Thirty Rules for Healthcare Leaders

Thirty Rules for Healthcare Leaders

Sanjay Saint, MD, MPH
Vineet Chopra, MD, MSc

Published in the United States of America by
Michigan Publishing

ISBN 978-1-60785-541-5 (paper)
ISBN 978-1-60785-542-2 (e-book)

To my wife, Veronica Saint,
the most inspiring leader I know
—Sanjay Saint

To my parents, Inder and Nanita,
who taught me to lead from the heart
—Vineet Chopra

TABLE OF CONTENTS

Foreword (Sachin H. Jain, MD, MBA, FACP)   ix
Preface   xiii
Acknowledgments   xv

Introduction   1

RULES

1. Hire Hard   5
2. Forge the Followers You Want   9
3. Try a Stress Buster   13
4. Watch Your TLR   17
5. Beef Up Your EQ   21
6. Know When to Be Tight—or Loose   25
7. Forgive and Remember   29
8. Don't Forget You Are a Role Model   33
9. Remember the Tree-Climbing Monkey   37
10. Counter the Constipators   41
11. Cultivate Effective Mentors   45
12. Develop Effective Mentees   49
13. Avoid Mentorship Malpractice   53
14. Write It Down   57

15.	Make a Friend before You Need One	61
16.	Smile Early and Often	65
17.	Motivate Change from Within	69
18.	Watch the Clock	73
19.	Let Data Set You Free	77
20.	Embrace Difficult Conversations	81
21.	Encourage Disagreement; Discourage Conflict	85
22.	Positive Deviance Is Your Friend	89
23.	Use Stress to Enhance Performance	93
24.	You Create the Culture	97
25.	Pursue Profound Simplicity	101
26.	Know When and Where to Draw the Line	105
27.	Patience Is a Virtue	109
28.	Negotiate with the End in Mind	113
29.	Don't Forget Family	117
30.	Lead with Kindness, Compassion, and Love	121

Appendix: Guide to Key Leadership Books	125
Additional Readings	131
About the Authors	143
About the Artist	144

FOREWORD

Over the last decade, there has been a pronounced growth in interest in management and leadership training for physicians. The reason is simple. We need people who can fix our broken healthcare system. The competencies expected of new physicians and change leaders include the ability not only to deliver high-quality clinical care but to effectively operate and lead within increasingly complex organizational constructs. And yet, only a small fraction of physicians receive any type of formal training in management and leadership.

A growing number of MD-MBA programs and medical school and residency tracks have emerged to fill the void. Realistically, however, barring a massive reorganization of medical education to emphasize the primacy of leadership and management skills, the availability of such training far outstrips the demand and, more importantly, the need. Also, doctors in the workforce who now have day jobs and patients who depend on them have few venues in which to gain the skill and perspective they need to lead.

Enter Drs. Saint and Chopra.

Their book—replete with pithy lessons that draw from practical wisdom and rich experiences as frontline leaders in American medicine—presents the management and leadership lessons that are most relevant to physicians as they try to drive performance, implement new programs, and guide others toward a common vision. These are not lessons from amateurs or self-proclaimed "gurus" or "visionaries" but from bona fide leaders of our profession—passionate medical educators and mentors with deep experience driving improvements in healthcare quality. The messages they present are timely and practical. They recognize the thorny, real-world obstacles that stand in the way of change. And they don't sugarcoat the analysis and the solutions. They avoid the highly saccharine quality of many purported leadership books and tell the reader "how it is." In this way, this book is a rare gift of authentic guidance to the reader.

Some of these lessons contained herein will make immediate sense to the reader. They draw on common scenarios we all face. And others, depending on the stage of one's career, will be filed away for use sometime in the future. There is not a single lesson that, over the course of one's career, won't one day be relevant to an individual trying to drive change or make a difference in a profession, industry, or world that desperately needs changing.

Early in my own career, I sought mentors who encouraged me. As I progressed, I was more interested in people who told me the truth about how the world works and gave me the critical feedback and skills I needed to make a difference. Over time, this book can become the kind of leadership bible that will prompt and inform the real conversations and discussions between mentors and mentees that we desperately need. We need to talk turkey about why change is hard and make it easier for trainees and emerging change leaders to understand.

My own small contribution to the message of this book, drawn from experiences working in frontline care delivery, government, the pharmaceutical industry, and managed care, is to urge the reader to hold on to his or her courage and maintain strongly held convictions. The pressure to conform is sometimes strong and invisible. It is easy to confuse "leadership" with toeing the company line, to pass the test that others have written.

More than anything, we need leaders who can call out contradictions and challenge the status quo, gracefully have the hard conversations, and make the hard decisions that need to be made.

Courage—more than ambition—will change the world. I wish you the best in holding on to your courage.

Sachin H. Jain, MD, MBA, FACP
President and CEO, CareMore Health
Professor of Medicine (Adjunct),
Stanford University School of Medicine

PREFACE

We enjoyed writing this book. It represents an accumulation of kernels of advice we have received during our years of clinical work. As healthcare leaders, we have now moved into positions in which we often are asked to dispense advice to those seeking guidance. The pages that follow represent the most important pearls of wisdom we have collectively accumulated. Just as they have for us, we hope they will serve you well in your leadership journey.

The rules in our book are meant to be read in one sitting or one at a time when you have a few minutes to spare. We suspect some rules will resonate more than others. Take, for example, rule 10, "Counter the Constipators." Several years ago, we introduced the term "organizational constipators" as a humorous yet apt description of why some hospital initiatives fail. Specifically, we found that there were some hospital employees who say the right things at meetings and appear to be supportive of new practices. Yet, their action or inaction in moving the initiative forward ultimately undermines their words. We call these people "organizational constipators." If you have some in your organization—and we suspect that you do—we provide some guidance on how to overcome them. There are 29 additional such rules, each of which come with strategies for effecting change.

We have no doubt that we have overlooked important points. Our intent was not to be exhaustive but rather to outline what we believe are the important tips that will help you become even more successful than you currently are. In other words, allow our hindsight to be your foresight.

Sanjay Saint, MD, MPH
Vineet Chopra, MD, MSc
Ann Arbor, MI

ACKNOWLEDGMENTS

This book would not be possible without the help and support of numerous colleagues and friends who have guided us on our respective journeys in healthcare leadership. Our own mentors and supervisors have influenced us more than they will ever know.

For Sanjay, this list includes Deb Grady, Larry Tierney, Warren Browner, Bob Wachter, Lee Goldman, Bill Seaman, Steve Fihn, Ben Lipsky, Bill Bremner, Walt Stamm, Rick Deyo, Tom Koepsell, Larry McMahon, Rod Hayward, John Carethers, Gil Omenn, Eric Young, Robert McDivitt, Grace Su, Mike Finegan, Carol Kauffman, Tim Hofer, and Jim Woolliscroft.

For Vineet, this list includes Erdal Cavusoglu, Mark Larey, Scott Flanders, Sanjay Saint, Larry McMahon, Bob Wachter, John Carethers, Rod Hayward, and Andy Auerbach.

We would also like to acknowledge our employers—namely, the University of Michigan and the VA Ann Arbor Healthcare System. Both are exemplary places to work, and we are fortunate to be faculty members and physicians at such superb institutions.

This book is the combined work of many individuals, and we greatly appreciate the assistance of Jasna Markovac, Jason Mann, Jason Engle, Rachel Ehrlinger, Michele Mazlin, and Laura Petersen.

We also thank our artists—Victoria Bornstein, Gina Kim, and Danny Suarez (all current or former students at the Penny W. Stamps School of Art and Design at the University of Michigan)—for each creating their own vision of what the art should look like for the three different versions of this book. When we posted an ad for an illustrator at the Stamps School, we had planned on hiring one artist. Our pool of candidates exceeded our expectations, and we narrowed down our selection to these three very talented individuals. We asked each of them to develop drawings for the rules and for the covers in their own style. The text in all three versions of the book is identical.

Finally, we thank our families for reading drafts of this work and for providing support and encouragement during our careers.

INTRODUCTION

Surprisingly little has been written about leadership in the healthcare setting. This is in part because of two widespread assumptions: first, that healthcare leaders can simply follow best practices designed for business leaders and be successful and, second, that they already have what it takes to be successful leaders.

Not so.

In *Good to Great and the Social Sectors*, the business consultant Jim Collins explains the basic difference between the business world and the world of healthcare: "In the social sectors [as opposed to the business sectors], the critical question is not, 'How much money do we make per dollar of invested capital?' but, 'How effectively do we deliver on our mission and make a distinctive impact, relative to our resources?'" Healthcare generally falls within the social sector.

This disparity of missions has led to different kinds of leadership best practices. CEOs of for-profit organizations, for example, can be confident that their decisions will be implemented provided that the result would be a positive contribution to the bottom line. However, healthcare leaders must learn to deal with a clutch of independent power bases, including tenured professors, physician leaders, nurses, administrators, volunteers, and a slew of allied health professionals. In general, these people do not enjoy taking orders, and they may not have a reporting line to the CEO.

The command-and-control leadership approach of many business leaders simply does not work in a healthcare setting. Healthcare leaders have to master other skills, particularly how to communicate, influence, and persuade. Often, they must inspire their personnel to go beyond their immediate self-interest to that of their teams or even that of their patients. This is no easy task.

As academic leaders and physicians, we, the authors, have decades of experience in healthcare and a sustained professional interest in healthcare leadership. In this book, we share healthcare-oriented best practices we have discovered during our research on the topic with the goal of providing tools and advice to time-pressured professionals in a useful and usable form.

How best to codify these principles? We thought back to our early days as house officers and fellows where we regularly felt overwhelmed by our responsibilities and the limited hours to fulfill them. And we remembered how grateful we were to those supervising physicians who would give us short, bite-size nuggets of knowledge that were targeted to the particular patient, case, or problem we were seeing. After all, no one had time for long, rambling lectures!

One of us recalls his surprise, and delight, when he learned from his attending that a patient's likely fungal infection could be narrowed down based on the first few digits of that patient's Social Security number. The attending explained that the first three digits indicate where the patient signed up for Social Security and different fungal infections favor particular locales.

These clinical aphorisms were certainly precious to us. And aside from their time-saving advantage, these axioms tended to have, as Mangrulkar and colleagues put it, a "pithy, even catchy" delivery style, which "adds to the likelihood of recall."

In assembling our favorite rules for healthcare leadership, we attempted to include such short, relevant examples that help illustrate what we mean and will hopefully help you, the reader, gain from our experience. We also provide a list of references and additional resources to permit further study of the advice we are offering. And each rule has a quote that (hopefully) underscores the point.

According to Peter G. Northouse, there are two basic kinds of leaders: "assigned leaders" who have leadership responsibilities based on the position they occupy in an organization and "emergent leaders" who have substantial influence no matter their official position or title. Studying quality improvement initiatives in hundreds of hospitals over decades, we encountered both varieties. Some assigned leaders—managers, executives—played major roles in successful initiatives, while others offered little or no active support. Yet at some of the hospitals where the assigned leader support was the weakest, the initiatives were extremely successful because of the leadership of nurses and physicians on every bureaucratic level—the emergent leaders.

Our "rules" have been written to appeal to both kinds of leaders. And they are not just for those in management. We hope they will also speak to healthcare colleagues in nonmanagement positions, as we believe they may most benefit from them. As Bennis and Nanus wrote, "Managers are people who do things right and leaders are people who do the right thing."

We invite you to take a look at our rules. We hope you will find them both entertaining and useful. And we hope they will help you as much as they have helped us.

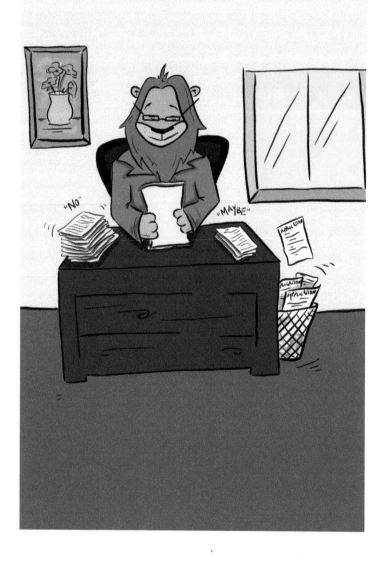

#1
HIRE HARD

When you lose a key staffer, you suffer. And because you are suffering, you want to find a replacement—fast.

Be warned: Healthcare leaders must learn to go slow when hiring. Yes, grab the candidate of your dreams. But if that paragon does not show up immediately, be patient.

Never settle for second best. Based on hard-won experience, we can tell you that once you hire soft, you are in trouble for at least three reasons. First, it is often difficult to remove an underperforming employee. Health organizations (especially universities or other public institutions) can be rigid that way. Union rules are even tougher. An infection prevention leader told us of waiting a whole year to fill a crucial vacancy before she found the right person. It was ultimately the right decision, she said, adding, "My life is so much better." Second, we tend to compensate for underperforming employees—often at great cost to others or ourselves. A charge nurse once told us, "I hired this person to help, but she ended up needing so much assistance that it was often easier for me [and others] to do the work. The environment quickly became toxic." Third, hiring the right people is the key to achieving success. In the words of Steve Jobs, "The secret of my success is that we have gone to exceptional lengths to hire the best people in the world."

Management guru Jim Collins writes: "The moment you feel the need to tightly manage someone, you've made a hiring mistake. The best people don't need to be managed. Guided, taught, led—yes. But not tightly managed." And what if you discover you have made a mistake? Most organizations have a probationary period during which laying off employees is relatively straightforward. This also applies to federal agencies and universities. Know what the rules are, and if you discover you made a hiring error, fix it before it's too late.

Hire hard, and in the long run, you will manage easy. One reality check here: Be realistic. While it is important to try to hire the perfect candidate, make sure your expectations are reasonable, that the ideal candidate does exist, and that you can afford them—a potential challenge, especially in public institutions.

> *"If you can hire people whose passion intersects with the job, they won't require any supervision at all. They will manage themselves better than anyone could ever manage them. Their fire comes from within, not from without."*
>
> —Stephen Covey

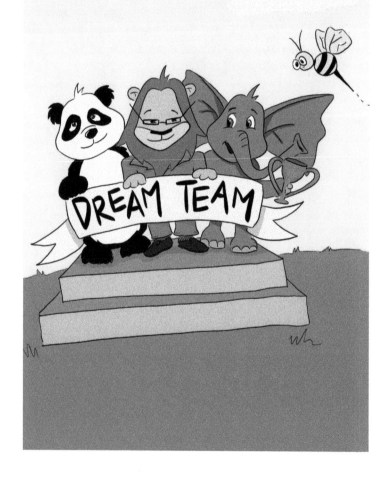

#2
FORGE THE FOLLOWERS YOU WANT

Until Robert Kelley came along with an article in the *Harvard Business Review* in 1988, management gurus paid little or no attention to followers—people who get the job done. Kelley suggested that serious thought be given to measuring and improving the performance of followers, which (at the time) was a management revelation. It remains a good idea not just in management—but in healthcare as well. (Throughout this chapter and book, we will use the terms followers, team members, and staffers somewhat interchangeably to designate the people with whom the more senior individual interacts within the hierarchy of their organization.)

You are striving for a dream team. Kelley's exemplary "follower" is still the gold standard. These are the people who are committed to their institution's goals. They manage themselves effectively, they constantly strive to improve their skills, they are innovative and independent, and they are willing to question their leader respectfully. In Kelley's words, they are "courageous, honest, and credible."

While these types of followers are ideal, they are hard to find. Craft your own team by moving your existing followers in this direction. As a start, sit down with each of your immediate reports and have a direct discussion about their responsibilities and your expectations. Ask them how they see their role on the team and then, if necessary, clarify what you expect them to accomplish. And in order to encourage your team members to rise to their potential, consider scheduling regular, one-on-one sessions to provide feedback and encouragement.

It is essential that you are clear about your expectations and tailor this to the team and individual. Your goal is for each team member to have an explicit understanding of how they will contribute to the organization's mission. You are already starting from a position of advantage, since most healthcare professionals are fully committed to the patient-centered mission. If physicians are part of your team, you can be fairly sure that they have a healthy sense of independence and will not hesitate to question you!

It is important to remember, as Kelley eloquently said, "Instead of seeing the leadership role as superior to, and more active than, the role of the follower, we can think of them as equal but different activities." That is an attitude that will go far in helping leaders get the kind of followers that they want and need. As a practical point, it may be best not to refer to your team members as your followers.

"A great person attracts great people and knows how to hold them together."

—Johann Wolfgang Von Goethe

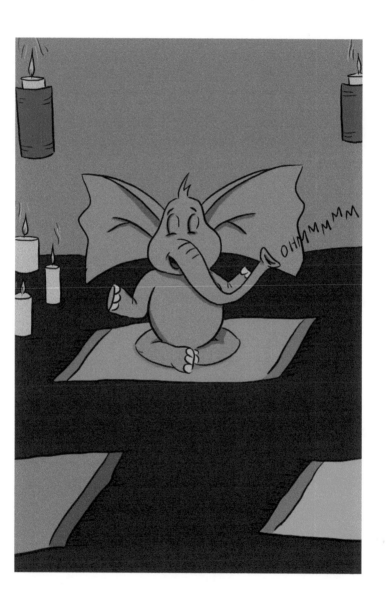

#3
TRY A STRESS BUSTER

In theory, stress is not a bad thing. The chemicals and hormones that are released when you confront danger prepare your body for fight or flight. But, if that stress response becomes a routine part of your life, it can cause headaches, depression, irritability, and a variety of chronic health problems. In healthcare, stress is the enemy of everything you work to achieve as an effective and positive leader: a cooperative spirit, a high level of efficiency, and a patient-centered, empathic environment.

Try a stress buster: the practice of mindfulness. A technique that has roots in Buddhism and yoga, mindfulness has been used with substantial success in hundreds of organizations, including medical centers. Mindfulness asks that you abide by the precept to "live in the present." You must learn to focus all your attention on what you are doing, without being distracted by other concerns. For example, when a mindful physician is with a patient, they are fully present in that room. They are not worrying about the latest email from the chief of medicine, their schedule, or an overdue credit card bill. Similarly, the mindful physician pauses to consider alternative diagnoses when reflecting on the cause of a patient's medical condition and remembers to perform hand hygiene before entering a patient's room.

The mindful state allows you to see everything afresh, with a beginner's mind. You learn to look at yourself in the moment. Are you giving the person with whom you are talking your full attention? Have you empowered them to express ideas and feelings? Have you discovered what they want from you and have you provided that?

Attractive as it sounds, mindfulness is no quick fix. It has to be learned and practiced. And that takes time. But perhaps not too much time: a review of the literature found that mindfulness exposures lasting four or fewer hours per week can improve healthcare provider wellness and patient care.

Mindfulness helps underscore the principle of equanimity: mental calmness in a chaotic situation. Or...what will be, will be—radical acceptance, if you will. We in healthcare often want to control every detail and aspect of care. We end up grasping. Mindfulness teaches us that this is impossible and counterproductive. Learning to slow down to pause, reflect, and see things afresh is not just good for you, after all. It is also good for patients whose care is entrusted to you.

"All things are preceded by the mind..."

—Siddhārtha Gautama

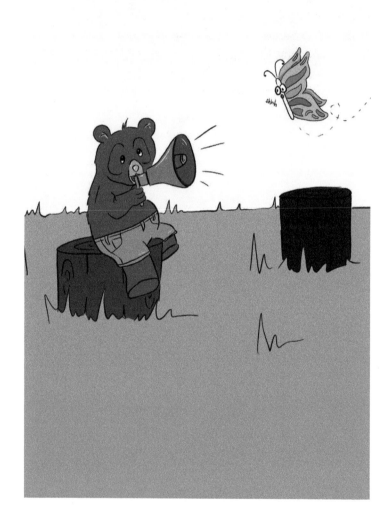

#4
WATCH YOUR TLR

Talking-to-listening ratio (TLR) is management-speak for a leadership pearl of great value, especially in a healthcare setting. By keeping track of how much you talk versus how much you listen, you learn how and when to keep quiet.

As Mark Goulston wrote in 2015, "There are three stages of speaking to other people. In the first stage, you are on task, relevant and concise...the second stage (is) when it feels so good to talk, you don't even notice the other person is not listening. The third stage occurs after you have lost track of what you were saying and begin to realize you might need to reel the other person back in." Rather than finding a way to re-engage the other person by giving them a chance to talk while you listen, "the usual impulse is to talk even more in an effort to regain their interest."

When you are talking, you are not listening—and when you are not listening, you are not learning. Executives who do all the talking at meetings do not have the opportunity to hear the ideas of others. Physicians and nurses who do all the talking are not discovering what patients want to say, or what potentially mistaken conclusions their students are drawing. They are also not hearing possible new approaches. The goal, then, is to ensure that your TLR is less than 1.

In addition to its value in monitoring your own talkativeness, the TLR can also be used to measure others. For example, when interviewing a new hire, apply TLR to discover how much patience would be required to work with the candidate. We once interviewed a physician whose TLR was north of 20...we passed on hiring them. If you find yourself in a situation in which you must work with someone with a high TLR, say over 5, what can you do? Our recommendation is to make an agenda (especially if the chatty one is your boss) and point to the agenda when the boss goes off on tangents. If the talkative one is a direct report or a colleague, remind them that you have another meeting in 30 minutes, so they will need to move things along.

The most surprising aspect to us about high TLR'ers is how oblivious they tend to be about the effect they have on people. Those with a high TLR usually remain that way.

"Better to remain silent and be thought a fool than to speak and remove all doubt."

—Abraham Lincoln

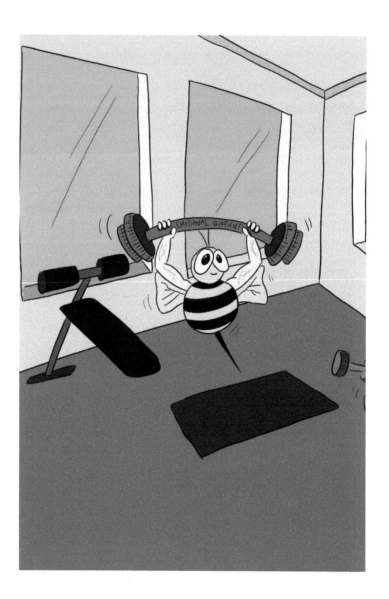

#5
BEEF UP YOUR EQ

If you want to bring change of any kind to a healthcare institution, you better wear your negotiating shoes and prepare to do some tap dancing. To ease your way, it helps to have a goodly helping of emotional intelligence, what is often called EQ (emotional quotient), as opposed to IQ (intelligence quotient).

As Don Goleman notes, emotional intelligence is the ability to understand your own emotions and those of other people and to use that knowledge to change the way you behave toward them. It is not simply a natural knack for sensing how others feel. It requires considerable assessment and adjustment of your own feelings and the way you manage them in your social interactions. "Your EQ is the level of your ability to understand other people, what motivates them and how to work cooperatively with them," argues the psychologist Howard Gardner from Harvard University.

EQ consists of several key components: self-awareness, self-regulation, empathy, critical interpersonal skills such as effective communication, and the ability to motivate others.

When one of your staffers comes in late to a meeting for the Nth time, you are likely to react with annoyance and/or anger that can impede your ability to be effective at the meeting. As Epictetus, the Greek philosopher who was born into slavery, wrote almost two millennia ago: "Any person capable of angering you becomes your master."

A high EQ enables you to pause and contain your immediate emotions. You may consider why the staffer is always late rather than dwelling on their latest episode of tardiness—and then address that question later, in a calm and private meeting. The result might surprise you (e.g., a marital dispute or family problems) and may help your employee feel more connected to you, underscoring the value of asking before judging.

Corporations and institutions all over the world offer classes to help improve EQ, and studies show the programs can be very effective. Inevitably, a lot depends upon how much time and effort you are ready to invest in the process. Our view is that IQ is a threshold function—you just need to be smart enough—while EQ is linear: the more of it you have, the more successful you will be. And, unlike IQ (which tends to be hard to change), EQ can be cultivated.

> *"When dealing with people, remember you are not dealing with creatures of logic, but with creatures of emotion..."*
>
> —Dale Carnegie

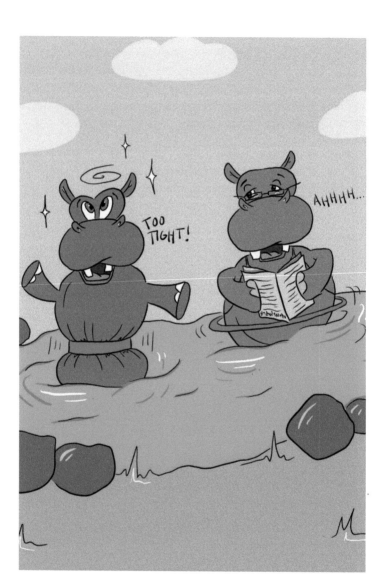

#6
KNOW WHEN TO BE TIGHT—OR LOOSE

The concept of loose-tight management was first introduced by Tom Peters and Robert Waterman in their 1982 book, *In Search of Excellence*. It has since been discussed and implemented in various forms by many organizations.

Generally speaking, there are **three domains** to pay attention to when managing someone:

1. Setting goals and expectations
2. Laying out the processes to achieve those goals and expectations
3. Holding people accountable to those same goals and expectations

For each of the above, the manager can be "loose" (i.e., implicit) or "tight" (i.e., explicit).

Far too many healthcare organizations are organized with a "loose-tight-loose" management style.

1. **Loose:** It is left to the employee to figure out what is expected of them to achieve the organization's goals.
2. **Tight:** Management closely controls the effort to achieve its goals. This is pejoratively known as "micromanaging."
3. **Loose:** Individual accountability is largely absent.

This is a formula for frustration, both for the team members and for you.

Most healthcare employees tend to be competent people. Unless your team is an exception, consider a different approach: a tight-loose-tight management style.

1. **Tight:** Define goals and objectives for success at the outset. Make it very clear to each person that they will be held

responsible for pursuing the goals of the organization and for meeting your expectations and standards.

2. **Loose:** Allow your team members to decide the best ways to achieve these goals—and stand ready to help them sidestep bureaucratic barriers.

3. **Tight:** Hold your people accountable for their efforts in pursuit of these goals and expectations, using reward and punishment.

If you are starting a new project, for example, you may have to modify things somewhat. We recommend more frequent meetings or brief calls rather than changing #2 above to "tight" (which is sometimes the tendency, since change often leads to anxiety and we therefore may resort to managing the details to alleviate our own anxiety). If you usually meet with your direct reports who are handling the new venture every two weeks, perhaps meet weekly until things are on track. They are still responsible for deciding the best ways to achieve the goals.

We have found that this management style helps teams feel engaged and empowered as you give people a chance to flourish. If done well, you will also flourish.

> *"Team members need to feel trusted and valued, and micro-managing communicates the opposite."*
>
> —Martin Zwilling

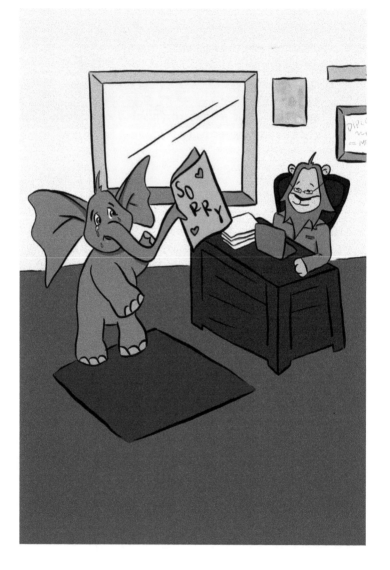

#7
FORGIVE AND REMEMBER

Mistakes and failures are inevitable. What is not inevitable is what happens next. Learning from mistakes and failures is the key to success.

As Robert Sutton in his 2010 *Harvard Business Review* article notes, great organizations learn from their failures and find ways to capitalize on hard-won experience.

In order to encourage learning, leaders must be willing to forgive. Forgiving implies a willingness to understand why a problem happened. Your followers are bound to make mistakes—that is part of growth in an organization, and you must always be prepared to deal with that. However, to forgive is not to forget—rather, every mistake should be viewed as a learning opportunity. Effective leaders seize on these moments to ensure that they don't happen again. That is, they forgive and remember.

Importantly, this rule applies to you. Forgiving themselves for making mistakes is something effective leaders must cultivate because it takes time. One technique we use when we make a mistake is reminding ourselves (and sometimes it helps to say this aloud) that we are doing the best we can, given the circumstances. This simple acknowledgment of kindness can help your mind relax and focus on learning from your mistake, rather than trying to put it behind you. Self-compassion is necessary in a leader…as is compassion for others.

Much as a person would prefer to forget making a mistake, forgetting is a surefire way of increasing the probability of the same thing happening again and again and again. Just as with medical errors, the "Forgive and Remember" approach allows for individuals and teams to become better. After all, remember Hanlon's razor: "Do not assume it is malice if it can be explained by simple incompetence."

When you forgive, you acknowledge that it is not possible for an organization to exist without mistakes. Forgiving recognizes that passing blame or judgment or holding a grudge creates a toxic environment and only makes you part of the problem. By choosing to discuss the error openly to learn from it, you can choose to forgive and remember. This, by the way, is the hallmark of highly effective organizations and teams.

> *"A life spent making mistakes is not only more honorable, but more useful than a life spent doing nothing."*
>
> —*George Bernard Shaw*

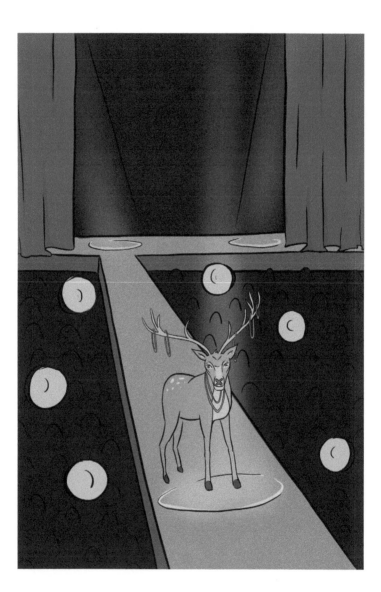

#8
DON'T FORGET YOU ARE A ROLE MODEL

As a leader, you are constantly being scrutinized. Every action or remark becomes a subject for discussion among your team members. You serve as a role model for most of your employees, whether you want to or not. Your ethical standards, your way of dealing with people and problems, and even your personal habits will be adopted, emulated, or criticized by your followers. In healthcare, that can be an overwhelming responsibility.

Nurse and physician leaders cope with daily periods of stress and frustration. If they lose their temper, that response will be discussed and met with disapproval. If they take risky shortcuts in their clinical roles, that behavior too will be noted and, all too often, adopted. We have witnessed the following several times: When the attending physician snaps at nurses or pharmacists, their medical students and residents think it is okay for them do that as well. When the attending physician forgets to wash their hands prior to touching a patient, so too will their charges. In the words of Darwin, like begets like.

We also see what happens when there is a change at the top. For example, the associate chief of psychiatry behaved in a condescending manner when his chief was also predisposed to condescension. When this chief was replaced with someone more collaborative and team-oriented, the associate chief followed suit. Examples of such shifts in behavior exist in many organizations across various sectors.

Similarly, healthcare leaders who model positive attitudes and responsible behavior can inspire their followers and those they encounter to do the same. One attending physician, a blithe spirit, told us that she was a "big believer in role modeling." She added, "There is a lot of joy-sucking that can happen in a hospital. It sounds trite, but I think you should just stop and smell the roses, and I try to make sure we pay attention to that."

Being a role model that your team looks up to will make it easier when you ask them to go in a different direction. As Gewertz and Logan wrote, "People's tolerance for change is strongly influenced by the level of personal comfort they have in their leader."

> *"Example is not the main thing in influencing others. It is the only thing."*
>
> *—Albert Schweitzer*

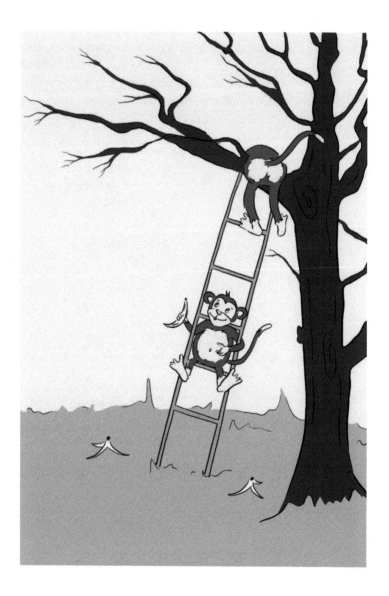

#9
REMEMBER THE
TREE-CLIMBING MONKEY

This rule is especially relevant for senior-level healthcare executives. Why? Because, the higher you go up the leadership ladder, the more you will be dissected in every domain. That is, the more of your bottom others will see. This is part of the territory. Once you become someone's "boss," you are no longer flying under the radar.

Simply put, every aspect of your behavior serves as a signal to those around you. For example, your facial expressions will be discerned as your liking what someone is saying or not. More people will laugh at your jokes than before (and trust us, you have not magically become more amusing after your promotion). And yes, more people will now read all kinds of meaning and hidden messages into those same jokes or off-the-cuff remarks. Every word, gesture, and communication takes on different meaning—leaving you exposed to misinterpretations like never before.

What's a good leader to do? First, be very careful of what you say and to whom. Assume that others will misinterpret any offhand comments. Second, pay attention to what you put into writing. We have seen many a problem arise from emails being misconstrued. This is especially true when a message is copied to many individuals, some of whom may not have the proximity to or context related to the subject matter. As a rule of thumb, if the issue is complex or nuanced—save it for a conversation rather than an email. And third, be careful of social media. You would be surprised at how many problems this may cause. Even posting a picture of yourself at a holiday party with a wine glass in your hand could be misinterpreted.

As is very often quoted in business settings, don't say, do, or write anything that you would not want to be seen on the front page of the *New York Times* or *Wall Street Journal*.

We have found the following rule of thumb useful: Resist the temptation to be funny or glib about a controversial topic. Errors tend to be acts of commission rather than omission.

In sum, people will pay more attention to you, your abilities, your demeanor, your honesty and integrity, your decisiveness, your mannerisms, and your attire. You are a leader now. Act accordingly.

"The higher the monkey climbs, the more you see of his behind."

—James Baker

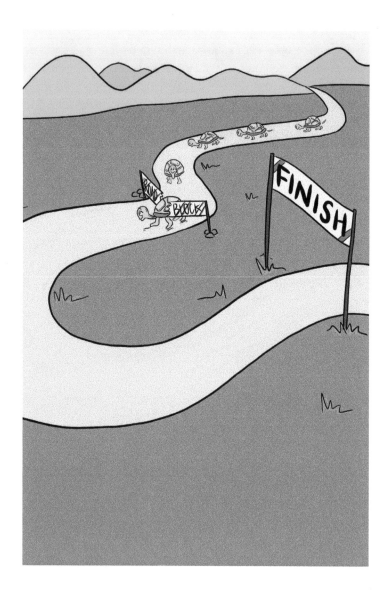

#10
COUNTER THE CONSTIPATORS

We used the term "organizational constipators" as a tongue-in-cheek description a few years ago in explaining why hospital quality improvement programs so often fall short. Our study found that the major culprits were the active resisters who openly opposed such interventions. But, there were also people who had no ill will toward the program; rather, they gummed up the works by their habitual management style. We call them organizational constipators, or OCs for short. You need to uncover them within your own organization—and take action to blunt their negative impact. OCs are like boulders in a river. If there is only one, the river flows around them. If there are too many, they dam up the flow.

There are two distinct varieties of these human roadblocks. The first enjoys exercising power. For example, we learned of a chief nurse who halted a second day of quality improvement training for one of her staffers. She said it was a "control issue" and disapproved of her underlings taking any action without her explicit approval.

The second gets in the way by doing nothing. Their inboxes and email accounts are overflowing with all sorts of urgent requests, including, for example, those to lift the hospital's performance quality. We all hear of administrators who put off signing purchase orders or delay new-hire approvals. Meanwhile, their supervisors, largely unaware, think these people are doing a good job, while their underlings cannot believe they still have one.

The OCs also damage your staff's morale and sour professional relationships. If you harbor any of them in your institution, take action.

One technique is to work around these people. For example, we know of a chief medical officer (CMO) who exhibited OC tendencies. His underling (the chief of medicine) wanted to conduct a quality improvement project and decided to tell his boss little about it. When problems arose, he simply went over the CMO's head to the hospital CEO. This can be effective in the short-term but does not alleviate the problem. And if the OC finds out—and they often do—there is trouble to be had.

Another technique is to reframe the OC's job description. For example, some hospitals let OCs keep their titles but rework their responsibilities so they cause as little damage as possible. Other medical centers wait until these people leave or retire.

A final—and perhaps best—approach for artfully dealing with organizational constipators is to use management jujitsu. We learned of this technique from a hospital CEO who cleverly convinced the OC that a new initiative was *the OC's* idea, thereby changing an impediment into a champion.

"There's daggers in men's smiles."

—*William Shakespeare*

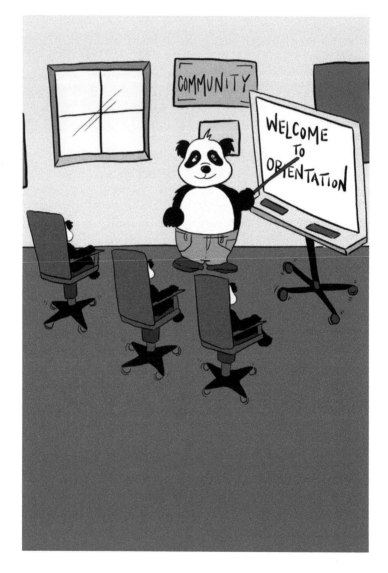

11

CULTIVATE EFFECTIVE MENTORS

Your institution runs on two essential kinds of relationships. The first is reflected in your organizational chart—who reports to whom all the way up to the CEO. The second is informal and uncharted and seldom occasions much discussion in the boardroom. It consists of the relationship between a wiser, more experienced staffer and his or her protégés—between mentor and mentees.

Successful mentors advance their own careers by developing those of their mentees. In doing so, they create a pool of loyal, high-performance employees. You have a big stake in encouraging mentorship because the more effective mentors you have, the more successful you and your institution will be.

Back in the days when staff, including faculty, used to spend their careers in a single institution, one-on-one mentoring made sense. But today, employees move from project to project and hospital to hospital. They need diverse skills and expertise that no single mentor possesses. And, with increasing time pressures, fewer hours are available for mentoring. That is why developing a team of mentors (so-called "mentorship teams") makes sense.

Mentoring need not take the form of a long-term relationship between a junior colleague and a seasoned expert—the traditional mentoring archetype. There are other archetypes to consider: coach, sponsor, and connector. A "coach" teaches people how to improve in a particular skill, such as doing a particular procedure or negotiating for a job. A "sponsor" uses their influence to make mentees more visible, recommending that a mentee serve on a panel or give a major talk at a meeting, for example. In so doing, sponsors risk their reputations when recommending junior colleagues. They, therefore, pursue high-potential individuals that are unlikely to disappoint. A "connector" is a master networker who serves to pair mentors, coaches, and sponsors with mentees. Malcolm Gladwell describes connectors as "multipliers that link us up with the world." To put it simply, the mentor guides, the coach improves, the sponsor nominates, and the connector empowers, but always the mentee benefits.

As a healthcare leader, you should not leave mentorship within your institution to chance. It is too important—and too often overlooked by management. Knowing that these archetypes exist and creating an infrastructure so junior staff can seek help will help your organization succeed.

> *"The delicate balance of mentoring someone is not creating them in your own image, but giving them the opportunity to create themselves."*
>
> —Steven Spielberg

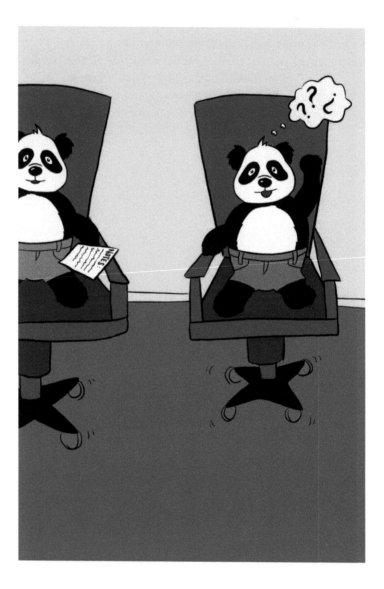

#12
DEVELOP EFFECTIVE MENTEES

While it is important to cultivate effective mentors, it is just as important to develop effective mentees. A highly effective mentee selects the right mentors; communicates clearly and efficiently; is engaged, prepared, and energizing; finishes tasks ahead of schedule; and plays well with others.

Our November 2017 article in the *Harvard Business Review* presents six habits ideal mentees should develop.

1. **Clarify what you need.** In identifying a mentor, you first need to decide what exactly you are looking for, what kind of support you need, and what your short- vs. long-term goals are. Do you need a sponsor, a coach, or someone who will help build your network and make connections for you?

2. **Choose wisely. It is essential to find the right person.** Your professional success and satisfaction are greatly impacted by your choice. Make sure that you can relate to your mentor and that their goals and their personal and professional attributes match your own. Your mentor does not necessarily need to be the most senior person you can find—sometimes they should not be.

3. **Underpromise and overdeliver.** Don't forget that mentors want closers—people who finish what they start. Learn to underpromise and overdeliver. This will serve you well, not just as a mentee but also in your professional career.

4. **Mind your mentor's time.** Mentors are busy people and tend to manage their time efficiently and wisely. They juggle and multitask. Be respectful of their time. Come to meetings prepared and set goals (and an agenda) beforehand. Send short, concise emails, with questions that require yes or no answers when possible.

5. **Beware of pitfalls.** Learn to manage up and guide your mentor. If mentors begin to malpractice (see next Rule #13), read the tea leaves and be ready to take action. If your mentor becomes a bottleneck, set deadlines with clear next steps. If your mentor starts to take credit for your ideas, more drastic steps might be warranted, including potentially finding another mentor. With a little foresight, missteps on both sides can be avoided.

6. **Be engaged and energizing.** Great mentees are fun to work with and mentors are much more likely to respond positively to them. When problems arise, and they will, don't just complain. Come with solutions and ask for guidance on which path is best. Use problems as a growth opportunity. When things do go wrong, accept constructive criticism and feedback. Remember, it is not personal, and you will grow from it.

"Tell me and I forget, teach me and I may remember, involve me and I learn."

—*Benjamin Franklin*

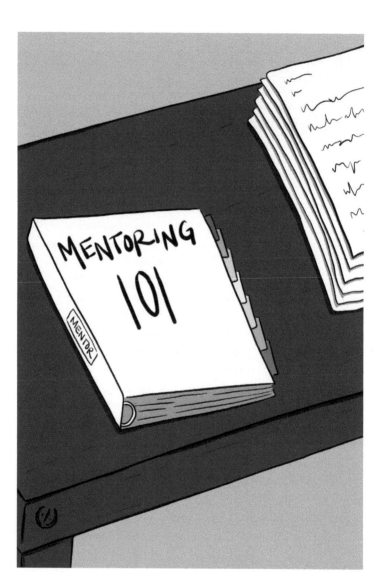

#13
AVOID MENTORSHIP MALPRACTICE

Much has been written about how to be a good mentor. However, there is little information about behaviors that make for a bad mentor. Because mentees are more vulnerable in the relationship, they must watch out for "mentorship malpractice." Part of the job of a leader is monitoring the mentoring experiences of the junior people in the organizations. When it comes to mentorship malpractice, there are two types to look for: active and passive.

A. Active Mentorship Malpractice

This form of malpractice is usually easy to spot because it is blatant. For example, a mentor takes credit for the mentee's ideas, projects, or funding. And the mentee can be an unaware participant, willingly giving up "ownership." Or, a mentor sabotages the mentee's success by giving them low-yield or nonacademic tasks or activities (e.g., becoming involved in projects that will not benefit the mentee or even running personal errands for the mentor). These types of behaviors often call for terminating the relationship. Your job as leader is helping the mentee find someone new (who is ideally an experienced, trustworthy, and successful mentor).

B. Passive Mentorship Malpractice

Marked by inaction on the part of the mentor, passive malpractice is gradual, more subtle, and harder to recognize. For example, the mentor stalls projects by being "too busy" to deal with what is expected, thus becoming the bottleneck in moving things forward, and the mentee's productivity suffers. Or, a mentor could be so averse to any kind of conflict or confrontation that difficult, but necessary, conversations or negotiations do not happen. Finally—and this is quite common in academic medicine—the mentor may be too busy traveling the world to spend quality time with the mentee. Though annoying, these types of behaviors are not necessarily deal-breakers. Mentorship teams, frank conversations, and alternative forms of communication (texting, Skype calls, or regular phone conferences) can salvage these relationships.

As can happen with any work relationship, the mentor-mentee relationship can stall or derail. Communication can break down or various work-related circumstances start to interfere, causing problems in the relationship. Your job as a leader is to ensure that the mentors in your organization do not commit serial mentorship malpractice. You should also help the mentee overcome issues and solve problems when they arise.

"Only the foolish would think that wisdom is something to keep locked in a drawer. Only the fearful would feel empowerment is something best kept to oneself, or the few, and not shared with all."

—Rasheed Ogunlaru

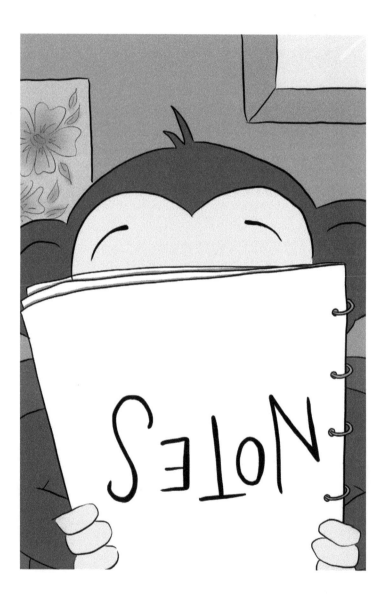

#14
WRITE IT DOWN

During a staff meeting or some other team gathering, how many times have you asked one of your people to take on a task, only later to find that the task remained undone? Did you say "infinite"? Sometimes, of course, the staffer remembered what was asked and decided to ignore it. But more often, they just forgot it because they had not written it down. The old Chinese proverb got it right: "The palest ink is better than the best memory."

Write things down. Creating lists of "to-dos" is such a simple solution, but it is so often overlooked. The next time you call a meeting, consider adding this to your email:

> Be sure to bring a pad and pencil (or electronic device) so you can make a note of any new tasks you are assigned or any new changes in how we do business. That way we can all do a better job of following through on things. (I will bring my own pad and pencil too.)

Keeping notes on what is expected should be part of everyone's routine. When we take part in external meetings, we pay attention to see whether the attendees are notetakers. It is a good indication as to whether the action items and decisions will be fully implemented.

As Paul Axtell suggests in his 2015 article, in order to ensure that productivity does not end after you walk out of the meeting, send out clear, concise notes, action points, and commitments that were made during the meeting. Alternatively, ensure someone on your team does this—but let them know they are responsible for this activity before the meeting starts.

We do this ourselves: One of us walks around from meeting to meeting with a composition book in which all the notes are in one place and to-do items are highlighted by an empty box that requires checking it off—a checklist of things to do.

> *"We don't like checklists. They can be painstaking. They're not much fun. But I don't think the issue here is mere laziness....It somehow feels beneath us to use a checklist, an embarrassment. It runs counter to deeply held beliefs about how the truly great among us—those we aspire to be—handle situations of high stakes and complexity. The truly great are daring. They improvise. They do not have protocols and checklists. Maybe our idea of heroism needs updating."*
>
> —*Atul Gawande*

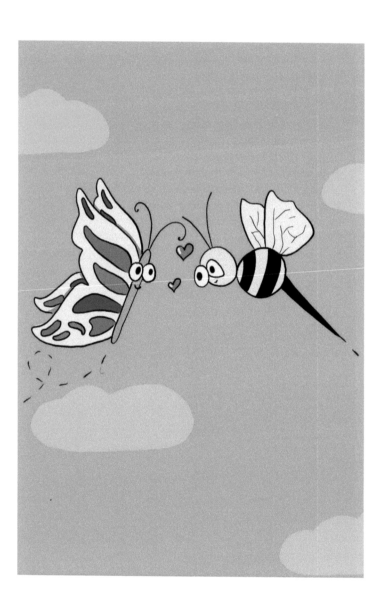

#15
MAKE A FRIEND
BEFORE YOU NEED ONE

To succeed in a hospital, leaders need a generous supply of social and political capital. This does not accrue overnight. Healthcare leaders need to make an everyday investment of goodwill and friendliness with those they encounter. The dividends may be slow in coming, but they are substantial and sustained. Friends give you the benefit of the doubt and help you when you are most in need.

Having friends (or friendly colleagues) at work is beneficial both professionally and personally. The benefits of social interactions have been studied for years and even more so in recent times, with the dramatic increase in the use of handheld devices. Eye contact between casual acquaintances passing each other in the hallway is replaced with eyes focused downward on smartphones. The result? We are becoming more socially isolated. Our personal solution? When we see professional colleagues (or patients and families in the hallways of our hospital), we nod in acknowledgment with appropriate eye contact and say hello. Even if we don't know them. You get a gold star if you remember the names of the professional colleagues you see frequently in the hallways or around the hospital.

We share an example from a search for a new department chair. The dean went on reverse site visits to meet the two finalists in their home institutions and asked them for tours of their hospitals. Candidate A walked around and it seemed like everyone knew her. She smiled and said hello to the people she came in contact with during the tour. Not so for candidate B—just the opposite. Guess who the dean hired?

Put away your phone, interact with your colleagues, and learn to make small talk—and not just with your supervisors or peers. Chitchat is an important "social lubricant," fostering a sense of community and teamwork. It helps bring down the divides that come from organizational hierarchies. It helps endear you to your staff.

Developing a reputation as a nice person who is quick with a smile and even quicker with a "good morning" pays off in the end. This reputation also makes it easier to give bad news, something that all leaders must do at some point.

> *"Takers believe in a zero-sum world, and they end up creating one where bosses, colleagues and clients don't trust them. Givers build deeper and broader relationships—people are rooting for them instead of gunning for them."*
>
> —*Adam Grant*

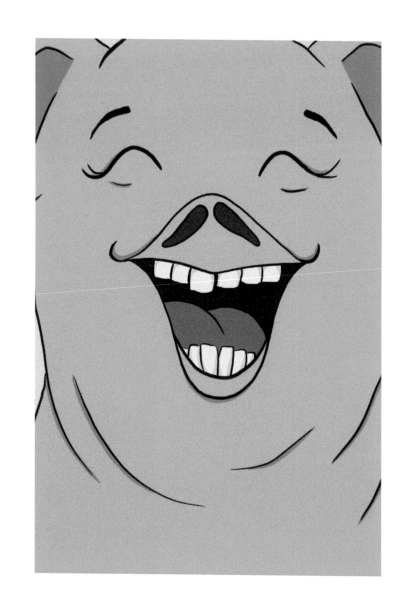

#16
SMILE EARLY AND OFTEN

Healthcare leaders must often inspire followers to their way of thinking rather than simply ordering them about. In his monograph *Good to Great and the Social Sectors*, Jim Collins distinguishes executive leadership from legislative leadership. Executive leaders have sufficient concentrated structural power to simply make decisions which are then followed. Legislative leaders, however, rely heavily on convincing their colleagues about the right course of action. Healthcare leaders are usually legislative leaders in that they must create the proper conditions for their preferred decision to occur. They simply cannot just issue commands. Your smile is an important ally in that process. It encourages collaboration and engagement.

In a previous book, *Teaching Inpatient Medicine*, we conducted an intensive study of 12 outstanding attending physicians, observing them on rounds and interviewing them, their current learners, and some of their past learners. One of the most noticeable characteristics of these exemplary clinicians was that they smiled a lot.

When these physicians entered a patient's room, they smiled. When they interacted with their learners, they smiled. And in both settings, we saw how their smiles got the encounters off to a positive, friendly start and helped them establish trusting relationships.

In general, their default demeanor was a smile. Even when their mouth wasn't actually smiling, they were smiling with their eyes. It helped them connect with patients, families, students, and colleagues. We suspect such behavior can be cultivated.

The physiology of a smile makes it easy (and pleasant) for us to do. When we feel happy, the body produces endorphins that cause our facial muscles to respond with a smile. That sends signals indicating happiness back to the brain. This feedback loop means that even when you "fake" a smile, you automatically improve your spirits, which in turn makes your smile more genuine.

One of us sets a personal goal on ward rounds—and that is, that at least once, the entire team must laugh. Similarly, we know of one healthcare leader who has instituted the following rule in their hospital: If an employee is within eight feet of another person in a hallway, for example, they smile and nod their heads to acknowledge the person is there. Within four feet, they say "hello" or "good morning." Try it. It is contagious.

"Kind words can be short and easy to speak, but their echoes are truly endless."

—*Mother Teresa*

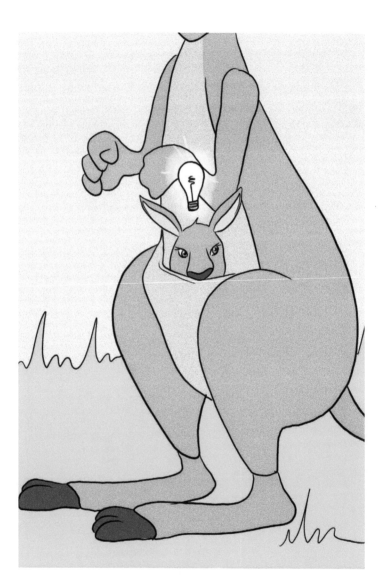

#17
MOTIVATE CHANGE FROM WITHIN

What can you do when some of your hospital's staffers—doctors, nurses, psychologists—are less than positive about a quality improvement program or refuse to accept evidence-based changes in the way they do their jobs? An effective solution can be to use a counseling approach that has been successfully applied to reluctant patients, probably by some of those very doctors, nurses, and psychologists.

This approach is called motivational interviewing, and it is being adopted by more and more medical centers around the country and the world. The technique is used to lead patients—for example, smokers and couch potatoes—to alter unhealthy lifestyles.

Motivational interviewing is collaborative rather than directive—the person doing it does more listening than talking and guides the other person to recognize how their actions may violate their own values. The goal is to help individuals see the discrepancy between what they want and what they are doing. In this way, the motivational interviewing practitioner helps the patient resolve this tension and move in the direction of accepting change. It is the opposite of instructing a patient to quit smoking or to exercise more. Such commands will elicit the "righting reflex" in which patients come up with reasons to continue their unhealthy decisions and stick to their guns.

As William R. Miller, the founder of motivational interviewing, has said, "Motivational interviewing is a collaborative conversation style for strengthening a person's own motivation and commitment to change."

To employ motivational interviewing as a healthcare leader, use two steps. First, ask open-ended questions to elicit information about current behaviors and feelings about changing or not changing those behaviors. By listening carefully to responses, you can restate views back to employees without judgment, moving the conversation in the direction of change by emphasizing statements about desire or intention to change ("change talk") while de-emphasizing "sustain talk"—statements about barriers or status quo. Second, ask your employee permission to bring new information into the conversation, something that will help illustrate why the change would be a positive one. In this way, the employee, in time, will decide on their own to wash their hands every time before touching patients or to withhold unnecessary antibiotics in patients with a viral infection.

"People are the undisputed experts on themselves. No one has been with them longer, or knows them better than they do themselves."

—*William R. Miller*

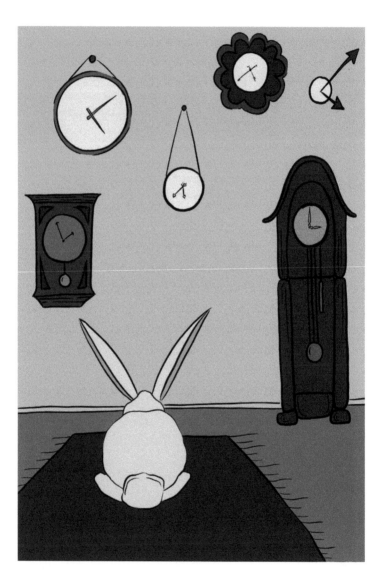

#18
WATCH THE CLOCK

Time is the most valuable asset for a healthcare leader. Quite simply, it is irreplaceable. Do not underestimate how valuable time is to your staffers.

We know leaders who always show up on time (or early) for meetings with their bosses or other higher-ups but not for their direct reports or other underlings. This "selective tardiness" is noticed by everyone. We know other leaders who are about 10 minutes late…always. When they do arrive, they apologize and make a weak excuse about why they are late. Take our advice: Do not be this type of leader.

Effective leaders start on time and finish on time. Not only does this keep work on track, but the practice also respects the time of others. Show up when you are scheduled to be there, and if you have a good reason to be late, let the people who are impacted know as soon as you can so they can adjust their schedules accordingly.

Keep meeting length to a minimum. Consider this: Why should you have a 30-minute meeting when a 15-minute one will do? Or, why have a 15-minute meeting if a 5-minute one will do? Don't meet for 30 minutes when you can meet for 20. As Victor Lipman asks at the beginning of his 2013 *Forbes* article, "Have you ever heard anyone complain a meeting was *too short*?"

Have an agenda (perhaps with time allocations) and stick to it. Do not go off on a tangent or let others digress away from the agenda points. If longer conversations need to take place about something specific, have those occur outside the meeting and report back at a subsequent meeting. Once two participants have three exchanges that do not include anyone else, it's best to table that topic and ask the two to meet separately and discuss.

Make sure you prepare before meetings and encourage your people to do the same. Set a good example. This is especially important in the health sector where people you interact with also see patients. Efficient and productive meetings, kept as short as possible, allow those people to get back to the business of helping patients.

Pay attention to the minutes, and the saved hours will follow. And saved lives might potentially follow as well.

"Beginning of a great day begins a night before."

—*Sukant Ratnakar*

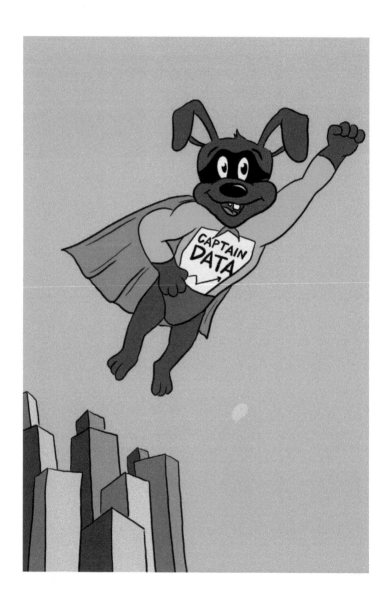

#19
LET DATA SET YOU FREE

Changing people's behavior is very difficult. It is easier to accomplish behavior change with cold, hard data. This is especially true in healthcare settings and when trying to modify physician or nursing behavior.

As Ray Williams pointed out in his 2010 post in *Psychology Today*, leaders need to understand and apply the knowledge learned in behavioral psychology and the lessons from brain science to effect organizational change. The reality is that organizational change will not happen without the people in the organization changing their thinking and behavior. Staffers will change their behaviors only if they understand the point of making the change and agree with it. This is where data can set you free.

Let us use an example we are exquisitely familiar with: a unit that is underperforming in removing unnecessary urinary catheters and thus has a higher rate of catheter-associated urinary tract infection (CAUTI) than it should. First, you must convince people that there is a problem. A powerful way to do this is to demonstrate that processes of care—proportion of unnecessary urinary catheters, for example—or outcomes, such as CAUTI rates, are worse than the benchmark (or expected) rates. Next, highlight how there is a gap between what should be done—ideally based on high-quality evidence published in a peer-reviewed journal—and what is currently being done in that unit. In our example, a unit may not have any system to ensure catheter removal even though a urinary catheter reminder system or a nurse-initiated discontinuation system are examples of what should ideally be used. Finally, once the intervention is implemented, provide follow-up data on processes and outcomes to demonstrate improvement.

Providing such follow-up data also allows for comparisons of different units, resulting in some healthy competition. After all, no one likes to be second best—especially in healthcare.

If you are having trouble getting started on an initiative in your hospital because of pushback from various employees, consider framing the change as a "pilot" rather than a new program. Who is against at least trying something that could help patients? Within that pilot, embed cold hard data gathering. The findings might help usher in the change you want to bring.

"In God we trust, others must provide data."

—Edwin R. Fisher

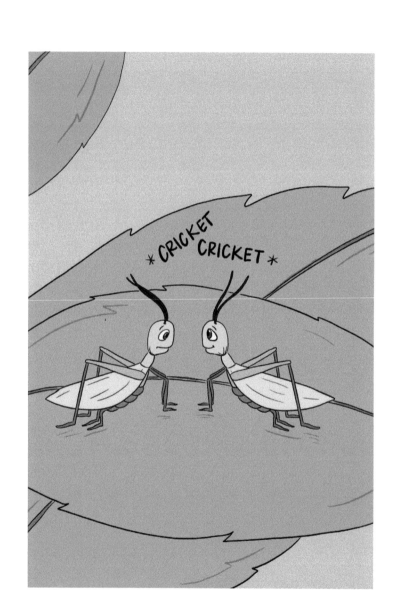

#20
EMBRACE DIFFICULT
CONVERSATIONS

Feedback is essential for the success of any team or program. Positive feedback is always much appreciated, but constructive criticism that prompts improvement is usually more valuable. It is not fair to expect your team simply to "know" that they are doing something wrong or something that is not aligned with your organization's or your expectations. They need feedback. Otherwise, how can we expect them to improve? If they are going down the wrong path, they will get to the wrong destination much faster if no feedback is provided.

These discussions in a healthcare setting are important and vital. However, discussions regarding inappropriate comments, preventable error, or ethical concerns are not just difficult—they are challenging. The temptation to avoid them is strong. Consider whether the conversation really does need to happen. Is the juice worth the squeeze? Oftentimes it is, but sometimes it is not.

If you decide to have the difficult conversation, it is your responsibility to ensure that it is as productive and helpful as possible. We recommend following the rule of thirds for these discussions.

It is usually best to start with what happened but spend no more than one-third of the conversation on this topic. You don't want to get bogged down in the past.

The next third of the conversation should be exploring how what happened made you feel and how the other person feels about the situation.

And then, the final third should be spent on figuring out with the person where you go from there. It is not enough to tell people what they are doing wrong; it is just as important, if not more so, to make suggestions about how they can improve. If possible, the constructive criticism should be part of a larger discussion that also includes things they are doing well. The message should be delivered kindly, privately, and without accusation or any personal affronts. The emphasis should be on the action (or inaction) and not on the person.

Your team may not remember all the things you tell them. They will remember how they felt when you talked with them. Effective leaders never forget the emotional angst of difficult conversations. While we believe candor is important, candor without kindness is cruelty.

Provide praise publicly and constructive criticism privately.

"Leaders relentlessly upgrade their team, using every encounter as an opportunity to evaluate, coach, and build self-confidence."

—Jack Welch

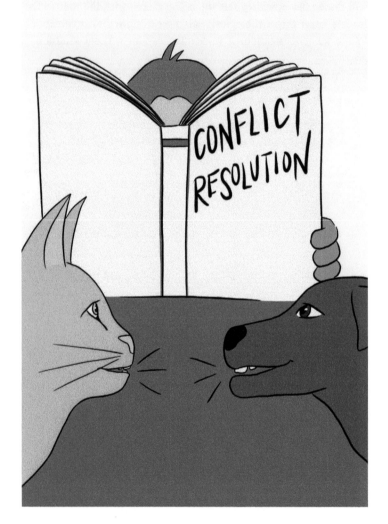

#21
ENCOURAGE DISAGREEMENT;
DISCOURAGE CONFLICT

Strong leaders know that not everyone will agree with their decisions. Rather than encourage a culture of silence, they welcome opinions of dissent and explore the reasons behind these differences as a means to learn and grow. Effective leaders, however, avoid outright conflict. The distinction is that conflict is not helpful, but productive disagreements can be. Effective leaders want the latter, not the former.

To illustrate, consider the following: One of us was leading a meeting where the number of shifts a faculty member would work at night was being discussed. The topic is contentious. No one likes to work nights, and worse, no one likes to be told that they have to do this—least of all physicians. One faculty member in particular was irate. Rather than ignore or dismiss this person's displeasure, the leader called on them, "I see you haven't said much, and you seem upset…would you mind sharing what you are thinking?" After hesitating, the faculty member spoke up: "I want to do my part, but I see people not working as many nights as others. If we are going to come up with a standard, shouldn't it be applied equally to all?"

The faculty member was right. Some faculty would not work as many nights as others—some for appropriate reasons, others not so much. A vigorous discussion ensued—one that was open and necessary. Had the leader not encouraged dialogue, this concern may not have been voiced, deepening a rift between faculty and leadership. When people feel as if they are unable to speak up and question their leaders, their concerns only fester and worsen. They may end up taking out their frustration in more extreme ways (e.g., leaving the position).

Another reason to encourage disagreement and discussion is to pressure-test decisions before they are implemented. If you are going down the wrong path, you will get there much faster if no one says anything. John Stuart Mill wrote, "He who knows only his own side of the case knows little of that." Disagreements ensure more than one side is considered.

During these conversations, it is important to be disciplined. We try to remember the following during a disagreement: Listen as if you know you are wrong and speak as if you know you are right. We also pay heed to the words often attributed to Sir Isaac Newton: "Tact is the knack of making a point without making an enemy."

"Honest disagreement is often a good sign of progress."

—*Mahatma Gandhi*

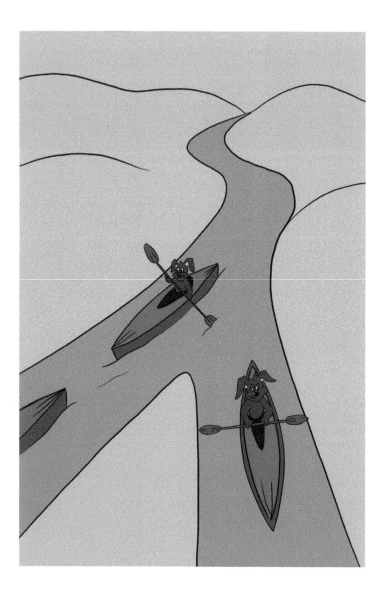

#22
POSITIVE DEVIANCE
IS YOUR FRIEND

To maximize the effectiveness of your team, find the bright spots, and make them work for you.

Positive deviants are behavioral and social change savants. They use uncommon, but successful, behaviors to find better solutions to a problem than their peers, despite similar challenges. Think about it—every organization has good doctors and good nurses. Good units and bad units. Your job is to find the uncommonly good ones, find out how they became so good, and help diffuse their approach to others.

For example, we started a program that would recognize internal medicine fellows—those who are specializing in cardiology, oncology, infectious diseases, or another medical subspecialty—who provided extraordinary clinical care during a monthly rotation. It is important to note that while subspecialists in private practice are paid every time there is a new consult, fellows are not. A phone call from a resident physician or a medical student to a fellow asking them to see a patient represents more work without more pay.

The program was simple. Residents and students voted for the fellow who provided the best care and the best service. Only those on the front lines who interacted directly with these fellows were able to vote. The monetary reward was trivial—a $25 gift certificate to a local pie company. The nonmonetary rewards were large: recognition by departmental leadership, a certificate suitable for framing, and a brief congratulatory meeting with the chief of medicine. As a result, not only did the fellows who were recognized feel appreciated, but the behavior of all fellows improved. After all, a little competition is a positive thing.

In their 2010 book about the power of positive deviance, authors Pascale, Sternin, and Sternin provide real-life examples of how positive deviance has facilitated the reduction of childhood malnutrition, neonatal mortality and morbidity, and the transmission of antibiotic-resistant bacterial infections: "There is no shortage of places where PD [positive deviance] could help."

Great healthcare leaders are often positive deviants. People want to follow them because they trust, respect, and admire them. According to Hollywood executive Jeffrey Katzenberg, "By definition if there's leadership, it means there are followers, and you're only as good as the followers. I believe the quality of the followers is in direct correlation to the respect you hold them in. It's not how much they respect you that is most important. It's actually how much you respect them. It's everything." Finding—and then rewarding—positive deviants in your organization makes that respect tangible.

"Deviance is in the eye of the beholder."

—Anonymous

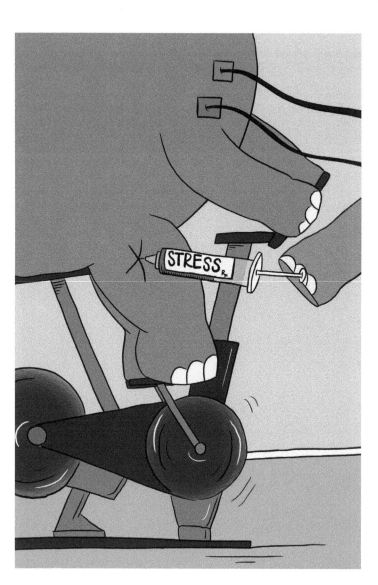

#23
USE STRESS TO
ENHANCE PERFORMANCE

Most medical students are taught the Frank Starling curve in Physiology 101. That inverted U-shaped curve with volume on the horizontal axis and cardiac output on the y-axis explains the performance of the heart based on the volume and stretch blood exerts on the myocardium. Too little blood, too little stretch—not enough cardiac output. Too much blood, too much stretch—and you have heart failure. If the stretch and blood volume are just right, you have perfect function and optimum cardiac output.

This physiologic principle applies as much to leadership performance as it does to cardiac function. In order to feel driven, leaders must learn to chase progress, pursue stretch goals, and learn to welcome change. In other words, feeling absolutely comfortable is not a position an effective leader should be in; effective leadership requires a moderate amount of stress at most times. In this way, new challenges that almost all healthcare leaders will encounter in their day-to-day activities—such as human resources-related problems or fiscal challenges—become a comfortable zone of performance. By embracing this discomfort, healthcare leaders also endeavor to expand horizons and anticipate what will be best for the organization down the road.

The relationship between stress and performance—moderate stress leads to maximum performance—generally applies to employees, mentees, and students. Indeed, effective leaders are so mindful of this relationship that they can titrate it so that each employee can feel challenged. For example, we regularly challenge our mentees to aim for higher journals or bigger grants—pushing them outside of their comfort zone.

Teaching on the wards is another example of this principle. When everyone is overly relaxed, little is learned and people become complacent. Conversely, too punitive an approach leads to fear—and no one learns when they are scared. Getting it just right—the right amount of stress that will optimize learning and patient care—is the goal. Great attendings do this by always being well-versed on their patients, knowing a bit more than their residents or fellows. This keeps the team on guard yet comfortable in doing their job. This is also what great leaders figure out how to do. If you have not already, we invite you to try it. The pressure might be just what is needed.

"Pressure makes diamonds."

—George S. Patton Jr.

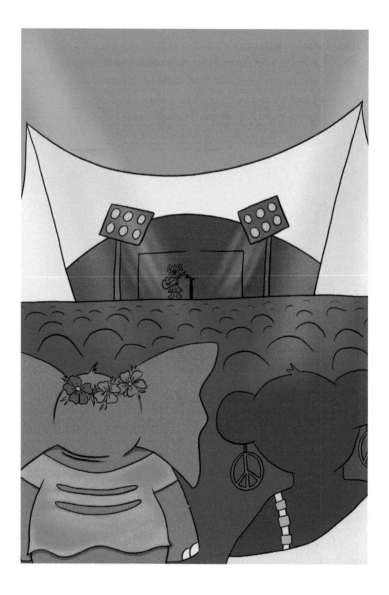

"The culture of any organization is shaped by the worst behavior the leader is willing to tolerate." This quote was making the rounds on social media in early 2015. It was presumably derived from a book on school culture, written by Steve Gruenert and Todd Whitaker and published earlier that year. The thing that made the quote resonate with so many people outside the education sphere is that it linked leaders to organizational culture. The implication is that if the culture is not good, the leader is to blame. And it is up to him or her to fix it.

As Garr S. Williams Jr. discussed in his LinkedIn post in 2015, leaders are not necessarily just the people at the top of the org chart. While every organization has its formal leaders, there are "informal" leaders—those individuals who are well known, respected, and listened to within the organization, regardless of their title or position. They do things that others do not want to do and often set the tone for those that work with and around them. For example, they take a stand, they speak their minds, and they do not put up with bad behavior. They address things head-on and, in doing so, represent the voice of an organization. These people are invaluable to a positive organizational culture. To be an effective leader, you must learn from these individuals. "Take a risk, have the conversation, and help lead your team to become all it can be!"

This will set the tone for the reputation your organization has both internally and externally. Your reputation as a leader and the reputation of your organization is what your employees (and patients for that matter) are saying when you are not present. And it is very obvious when staffers are not passionate about their work and organization.

It is up to you as a leader to decide what is and what is not acceptable behavior for your staffers (and also for yourself, as the role model). But always keep in mind that if you tolerate bad—or even less than great—behavior from individuals on your team, it will reflect on the culture of your organization.

As boss, you help shape your organization's culture by the things that you do—and don't do.

"For individuals, character is destiny. For organizations, culture is destiny."

—Tony Hsieh

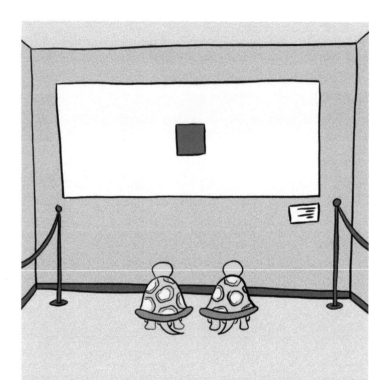

#25
PURSUE PROFOUND SIMPLICITY

Ralph Waldo Emerson once said, "It is the last lesson of modern science that the highest simplicity of structure is produced, not by few elements, but by the highest complexity." In what now seems clairvoyant, Emerson recognized that science often obfuscates truth with complexity.

In 1979, William Schutz postulated that learning develops in three sequential stages: (1) superficial simplicity, (2) confusing complexity, and (3) profound simplicity. In this model, a novice is typified by cursory explanations of complex processes, a product of nascent understanding. This is a necessary first step, but as expertise grows, confusing complexity—wherein intricate, elaborate explanations are offered for the process at hand—sets in. This is where much of the discourse in a field often exists (think experts debating concepts among one another). This is also a necessary step, since the emergence of profound simplicity comes from the ultimate insight that follows this discourse. Here, true mastery over a topic allows for the complex to be explained in terms accessible to most.

Here is an example: A hospital wants to improve upon the safety culture in their organization. Phase 1 (superficial simplicity) is when the CEO sends out an email to all employees stating, "We are going to improve the culture of safety. This is the most important goal of the year." We suspect that most employees glance at such emails and hit delete. Phase 2 (confusing complexity) ensues when there is discussion about what survey instrument will be used to measure safety culture, how differences among units or categories of healthcare workers (e.g., nurses vs. doctors) will be assessed, and how to *actually* instill a culture of safety. The final phase—profound simplicity—is the realization that we aim to treat every patient as if they are a family member, and that is how to create a culture that emphasizes safety.

The difference, in our opinion, between a good leader and a great one is the attainment of profound simplicity: mastery over a topic to such an extent that even the most complex can be made deceptively simple to those unfamiliar with the material. When you next run your meeting, think about how you frame arguments, define the vision, or create goals, then ask: Am I pursuing profound simplicity?

> *"Great leaders are almost always great simplifiers, who can cut through argument, debate and doubt, to offer a solution everybody can understand."*
>
> *—General Colin Powell*

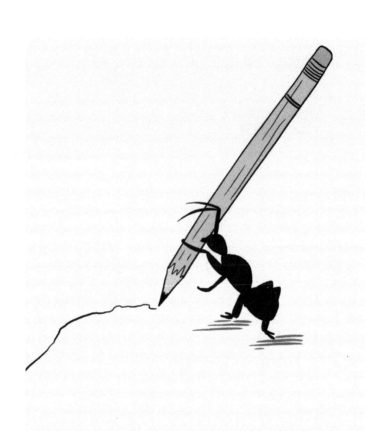

#26
KNOW WHEN AND WHERE TO DRAW THE LINE

Most of us spend more time at work or at activities related to work than we do at home. It is easy for professional relationships to blur with personal ones. Barring situations where work colleagues decide to pursue personal relationships outside of work, where does one draw the line? Is it okay to mix business with pleasure?

Your team members and your staffers will tell you about problems that affect their personal lives, the gossip about your colleagues, or even seek your advice about personal situations. While we all want to be sympathetic to these problems, it is important to maintain boundaries. You are not your staffer's unpaid therapist, their physician, or, for that matter, their close friend. You are their supervisor—responsible for their professional growth and that of your institution. Employee assistance programs and human resources specialists were created for these types of situations, not leaders like yourself. Effective leaders thus must learn to draw lines to preserve this distance. One need not be rude about this; a gentle "I'm sorry you are struggling with this. I suggest you speak with Anne in HR to see if she can help" is all that is needed to show that you care but cannot be the shoulder to cry on.

You can be close friends with people who are at a similar level in your organization—your "peer group." Those relationships can provide welcome support, since you may share the same boss or similar challenges such as hospital-wide budget cuts. These individuals can also serve as strong allies during leadership meetings when you may both advocate for additional resources for clinical services.

Keeping an appropriate distance also applies to the virtual world. The proliferation of social media blurs the professional and the personal. While organizations use social media to broaden their reach and to distribute their message, leaders must be careful to separate their opinions from the views of the organization. In particular, posting about your political leanings or controversial events should be avoided. Remember, items posted can last forever, even if you delete them.

Our rule of thumb before posting something on any social media site is to ask the following three questions (and post only if you have carefully considered the answers):

1. Is this helpful?
2. What are the downsides of posting it?
3. Whose feelings may it affect in a negative manner?

"Individuals set boundaries to feel safe, respected, and heard."

—Pamela Cummins

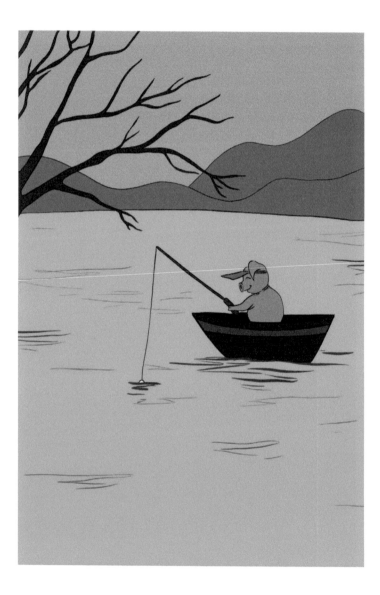

#27
PATIENCE IS A VIRTUE

Every physician learns the adage "Time heals all wounds." Just like healing takes time, so too does developing the skills you need to become a leader. Too many of us move from the world of clinical care—in which we have gained some expertise—expecting to easily transfer that clinical acumen into leadership knowledge.

Not so. While some of the lessons we learned as clinicians apply to our roles as healthcare leaders, there is much new terrain. And it will take time and patience to learn skills to survive in this new realm.

In their best-selling book *Learning Leadership*, James Kouzes and Barry Pozner provide a framework to help individuals to become the best leaders they can be. A key tenet of the book is that the best leaders are the best learners—and like most skills, learning leadership takes time. Whether it's recruiting, negotiating finances or budgets, managing difficult faculty or staff, or thinking about strategy and growth—it takes grit, resilience, patience, and deliberate practice to become a better leader.

Give yourself time to grow as a leader in healthcare. Take the time to invest in your leadership journey by taking, for example, week-long classes or executive education courses on management strategies. You should also read leadership books on your own or with others in healthcare. We started an attending physician leadership book club in which the attendings on one of our services were all given a series of books and took turns discussing these books during regular business meetings. Most of the readings came from outside of healthcare and included authors such as Malcolm Gladwell, Peter Drucker, Suzanne Gordon, and Jim Collins. The full list of books—with annotations—is available in the appendix.

Here is another way to improve: at the end of each workday, spend a few minutes reflecting on what went well today, why things went the way they did, and what you could have done better. Learn to be patient—not only with others but also with yourself. Just like those that report to you, you may not get everything right in the first place. You may well get more wrong than right at the outset. Taking time to grow, learning to get it right, and thinking about your leadership journey are the foundations to success.

After all, patience is a virtue.

"The two most powerful warriors are patience and time."

—Leo Tolstoy

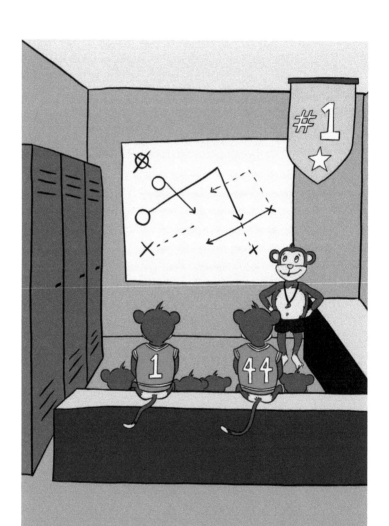

#28
NEGOTIATE WITH THE END IN MIND

Leaders negotiate—a lot. It is a skill they must learn early on during their tenure. Even when they don't realize they are negotiating, they are negotiating. They are negotiating with staff members who are considering joining the organization as well as with exemplary staff members who are being recruited elsewhere. Leaders are negotiating for resources for their department or unit and negotiating with underlings who are asking for raises or a promotion, more responsibility, or a more flexible schedule. Negotiation is core to being a leader. Healthcare is no exception.

There are two central kinds of negotiations: the one-time transaction, like buying a car, and the long-term commitment, like being in a relationship with someone. In the former, you want the best deal regardless of what happens to the other party. After all, it is your money and you are the buyer—you should get what you want out of the deal. You are unlikely to ever see that salesperson again, so hurt feelings are not a priority. In short, you leave nothing on the table. But in the latter scenario, the consequences of your decision matter because they are linked to events beyond that one single decision. They will affect the relationship you have with the other person for years to come. In other words, your decision is a part of a linked negotiation.

Effective healthcare leaders learn to negotiate with the end in mind. This means that they learn that give-and-take is part of the process. The best leaders know how much to give and how much to take. They negotiate with their eye on the end result and tend to take the long view, not with a single deal in mind. In other words, they understand that short-term loss may be needed for long-term gain.

For example, when negotiating to raise salaries for our faculty, we knew that give-and-take would be part of the process. So, we came prepared, preemptively agreeing to lower costs on one side of the balance sheet so as to provide some additional resources to our organization so that employee salaries could be raised. The result? We were able to provide physician salaries that were competitive in the marketplace and left the table feeling like both sides won. Similarly, when recruiting faculty, accommodating requests for protected time or travel support may help gain goodwill in the future. In linked negotiations, it is best to leave something on the table.

> *"The ability to see the situation as the other side sees it, as difficult as it may be, is one of the most important skills a negotiator can possess."*
>
> —*Roger Fisher*

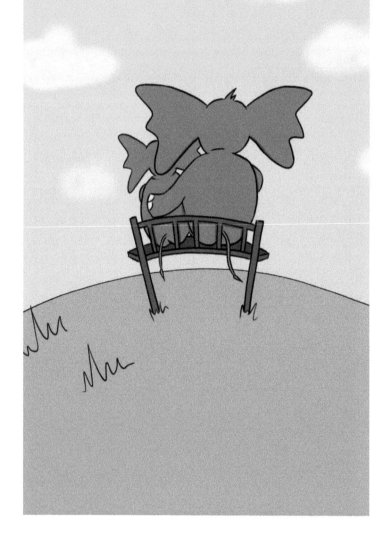

#29
DON'T FORGET FAMILY

Is it possible to devote the necessary time to family and loved ones given the pressures of the job? Yes. In fact, we think it is mandatory. When things are going well in your career, everyone will seem like a friend. When things head south and you face the inevitable hurdles, you learn who you can rely on. The people who have your back tend to be your family members. Make sure you don't forget them during the good times.

Our jobs make most of us unhappy at some point. The solution? Our families. Why? They—and other loved ones such as extremely close friends—provide us with a sense of purpose, connection, joy, and well-being.

But demanding jobs often take a toll on your personal life, in general, and your family life, in particular. When you have time conflicts and have to be in two places simultaneously—at a work-related presentation or your child's play, for example—what usually gives is your time with your children, since they cannot fire you. Unfortunately, they will be the ones adversely affected by the limited time you spend with them. You are replaceable at work. You are not replaceable at home.

We recommend two principles. First, try to be fully present when you are at home. This means limiting multitasking and putting phones and emails away—being fully immersed with those around you. Yes, you may need to work at home but do so when you are no longer needed by your children, your spouse, or other family. We operationalize this by using the opening of the garage door after a long day at work as our cue. As the door opens, we tell ourselves: it is now family time, so forget the last discussion you had with your boss or the presentation you have to give tomorrow. Bask in the love and laughter of your home, and do not take it for granted.

Second, stick to social rituals that allow you to connect to family and friends. Examples include family dinner every night with everyone around the table and no devices allowed. Or enjoying a regular meal (or coffee) with a close friend, going on after-dinner walks with your spouse, taking annual family vacations during which you are (mostly) off the grid, or playing family board games on Saturday night. You and your partner get to choose the family culture that you want to have. It is a choice you should make and stick with.

Leadership comes with professional and personal responsibilities. In the words of a colleague, "When you die, you will be remembered by many. Just make sure that some of them are your family."

"The most important thing in the world is family and love."
—*John Wooden*

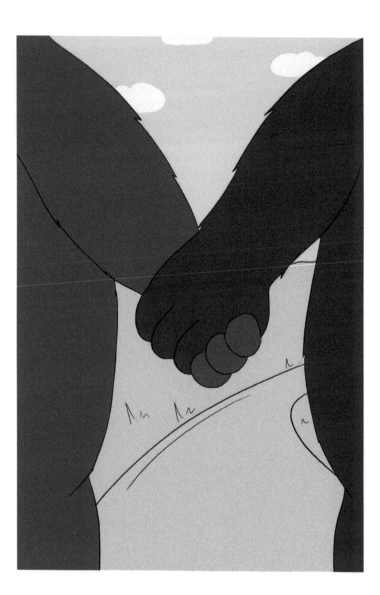

#30
LEAD WITH KINDNESS, COMPASSION, AND LOVE

Leaders today have been taught to lead with their heads, not with their hearts. They are expected to be rational, tough, and strategic so that they focus on the bottom line.

Yet, as Ray Williams posted in 2012, "Research on successful leaders and the current turbulent economic and social times calls out for a different style of leader—one that exhibits kindness, compassion and empathy." He gives examples of well-known leaders in charge of successful companies who were known for being combative, coercive, and purveyors of "smack talk" about their competitors and colleagues. These leaders, while successful from a financial perspective, were not ideal in the long run. Evidence shows that leaders who exhibit and value kindness at work, create a culture where people want to work. Not surprisingly, they are more productive than those who do not share these traits.

Kind and compassionate leaders communicate sincerely and openly. They are not rigid; rather, they are adaptable, flexible, and willing to bend the rules. Importantly, they do not criticize and judge others—they lead by example and pay attention to how their behavior is perceived by others. They are more leader than manager. As Bennis and Nanus said, "Managers are people who do things right and leaders are people who do the right thing."

When Avedis Donabedian, physician and founder of the study of quality in healthcare and medical outcomes research, found himself in the position of being a patient, he observed firsthand the problems in the healthcare system. He noted, "Systems awareness and systems design are important for health professionals but are not enough. They are enabling mechanisms only. It is the ethical dimension of individuals that is essential to a system's success." He went on, "Ultimately, the secret of quality is love. You have to love your patient, you have to love your profession, you have to love your

God. If you have love, you can then work backward to monitor and improve the system."

In healthcare more than in any other field, compassion and kindness for your patients, your colleagues, your leaders, and your followers are essential to your success. This, perhaps, is the most important rule of this book.

"Let us always meet each other with smile, for the smile is the beginning of love."

—*Mother Teresa*

APPENDIX
Guide to Key Leadership Books

Blanchard KH, Johnson S. The One Minute Manager. 1st Morrow ed. New York, NY: Morrow; 1982.

This book outlines the three one-minute techniques of a successful manager by using the anecdote of a young man in search of an effective supervisor. It discusses the importance of setting one-minute goals so employees can be aware of what's expected from the beginning. It emphasizes one-minute praises because they encourage and motivate staff to excel. Lastly, the one-minute reprimands discussed in the book involve informing staff of their errors but also reminding them how much they are valued.

Christensen CM. The Innovator's Dilemma: When New Technologies Cause Great Firms to Fail. Boston, MA: Harvard Business School Press; 1997.

Innovation is by its nature a disruptive process, shoving aside established products or protocols. But when that new product becomes the established product, stagnation can set in until the next disruptive innovation. Most companies fail to be their own disruptions, falling prey to the next upstart. Christensen examines the why and the how in this book, offering insight to those looking to remain exceptional.

Collins JC. Good to Great: Why Some Companies Make the Leap—and Others Don't. 1st ed. New York, NY: Harper Business; 2001.

Not all companies are formed with the best plans. This book examines the ways in which any company can transform from good (or not so good) into great, regardless of origins. Based on a five-year research effort, this book details some of the most surprising outcomes of looking at the best modern businesses.

Collins JC. Good to Great and the Social Sectors: Why Business Thinking Is Not the Answer. 1st ed. New York, NY: HarperCollins; 2005.

This monograph is a companion to the 2001 book *Good to Great*, intended to provide answers to reader questions specifically in the social sector of the economy. The work is based on interviews and workshops conducted with over 100 social sector leaders.

Collins JC. How the Mighty Fall and Why Some Companies Never Give In. New York, NY: HarperCollins; 2009.

Organizational decline is not inevitable, provided you have the right insight. Jim Collins explores in this book the reasons why organizations decline—even to the point of failure. He identifies five key stages of decline that must be avoided and asserts that being aware of these steps provides a chance for recovery and revitalization.

Drucker PF. The Effective Executive: The Definitive Guide to Getting the Right Things Done. 50th anniversary ed. New York, NY: Harper Business; 2017.

This book chronicles the best practices in management and leadership. It points out the importance of specific habits like time management, focusing on contributions to the group, mobilizing strengths, setting the right priorities, and making effective decisions.

Fisher R, Ury WL, Patton B. Getting to Yes: Negotiating Agreement without Giving In. 2nd ed. New York, NY: Penguin Books; 1991.
This book highlights an approach to creating sustainable negotiations called "negotiation of merits." The method is meant to allow both parties the opportunity to accommodate each other and foster a positive business relationship. The recommendations for this method involve separating people from the problem, focusing on interests instead of positions, inventing options for mutual gain, insisting on objective criteria, and knowing the best alternative to a negotiated agreement.

Gawande A. The Checklist Manifesto: How to Get Things Right. New York, NY: Metropolitan Books-Henry Holt & Co; 2010.
The author examines the use of checklists to reduce medical errors and improve medical and surgical outcomes. The book provides multiple examples of checklists reducing errors such as the implementation of the World Health Organization's 2-minute, 19-point Safe Surgery Checklist. Gawande effectively calls for the widespread adoption of checklists in the American healthcare system.

Gladwell M. Outliers: The Story of Success. 1st ed. New York, NY: Little, Brown; 2008.
This book studies an array of fields in order to uncover the key aspects of achieving success. The book looks at the benefits we are born with, examining factors that influence later success such as parental occupations, where you were born, and your upbringing. The book then focuses on learning about various ways people succeed and certain cultural legacies that have been influential.

Goldsmith M, Reiter M. What Got You Here Won't Get You There: How Successful People Become Even More Successful. 1st ed. New York, NY: Hyperion; 2007.

When comparing high-quality things, it can often be very challenging to discern which one truly is better. So it is with people too, especially when they have already achieved much. Some make it to that next level, though others never do. Goldsmith looks at the 20 bad habits that need to be broken to achieve that next level of success.

Gordon S. Nursing against the Odds: How Health Care Cost Cutting, Media Stereotypes, and Medical Hubris Undermine Nurses and Patient Care. Ithaca, NY: Cornell University Press; 2005.

The author examines how cost-cutting measures in healthcare have compromised quality of care. She also focuses on the workplace interactions of physicians and nurses and how negative stereotyping has devalued the contribution of nurses. Additionally, she calls for a new system that includes safer staffing, improved scheduling, and other policies that lend a stronger voice to nurses.

Heath C, Heath D. Switch: How to Change When Change Is Hard. New York, NY: Crown Publishing Group; 2010.

Change is hard. It never seems to come easily. This book brings together a diverse collection of research on the central, human conflict that often prevents us from adopting change. Using an anecdotal style, the authors present a pattern that can be applied to almost any circumstance.

Johansson F. The Medici Effect: Breakthrough Insights at the Intersection of Ideas, Concepts, and Cultures. Boston, MA: Harvard Business School Press; 2004.

Intersectional innovation—that particular kind of innovation that comes when people from different experiential backgrounds come together to fix a problem or create something new—is at the heart of *The Medici Effect*. This book offers insight into truly transformative innovation by looking at a diverse cross section of inspirational stories.

Kotter JP. A Sense of Urgency. Boston, MA: Harvard Business School Press; 2008.

In this book, the author determines the central obstacles toward changing a company and presents an eight-step process for business transformation. The first step involves highlighting the need to create a "sense of urgency" in order to combat all forms of complacency in a company.

Lee F. If Disney Ran Your Hospital: 9 1/2 Things You Would Do Differently. Bozeman, MT: Second River Healthcare Press; 2004.

When it comes to "outside the box" thinking, reframing the concept of healthcare delivery as an "experience"—rather than a service—is a true paradigm shift. In this engaging book, Fred Lee presents nine (and a half) principles that show how hospitals can be transformed into a beloved workplace and the destination your patients will always want to go for their healthcare.

Lencioni P. The Five Dysfunctions of a Team: A Leadership Fable. 1st ed. San Francisco, CA: Jossey-Bass; 2002.

In this book, the author explores the five major pitfalls that account for team failure in the business world. It uses a story about a struggling tech company and fictional team members to articulate its point. The factors which lead to dysfunction include absence of trust, fear of conflict, lack of commitment, avoidance of accountability, and inattention to results.

Topol EJ. The Creative Destruction of Medicine: How the Digital Revolution Will Create Better Health Care. New York, NY: Basic Books; 2012.

Genetic sequencing. Improved imaging. Smartphones. Big data. The author argues in this book that the revolution in healthcare is nearly upon us, as technology converges to allow for a level of personalization in medicine that has never been seen before.

Ury W. The Power of a Positive No: How to Say No and Still Get to Yes. New York, NY: Bantam Books; 2007.

Sometimes you have to say no. How you say it can have lasting impacts on the relationships you have. This book discusses methods in which saying no doesn't have to negatively impact that relationship and can, instead, lead to a positive outcome.

ADDITIONAL READINGS

INTRODUCTION

1. Collins JC. Good to Great and the Social Sectors: Why Business Thinking Is Not the Answer. 1st ed. New York, NY: HarperCollins; 2005.
2. Mangrulkar RS, Saint S, Chu S, Tierney LM. What is the Role of the Clinical "Pearl"? Am J Med. 2002;113:617-24.
3. Northouse PG. Leadership: Theory and practice. 8th ed. Thousand Oaks, CA: Sage publications; 2018.
4. Bennis W, Nanus B. The Strategies for Taking Charge. New York, NY: Harper Row; 1985.
5. Algahtani A. Are Leadership and Management Different? A Review. JMPP. 2014;2:71-82.

RULE 1: HIRE HARD

1. Bennis W, Nanus B. The Strategies for Taking Charge. New York, NY: Harper Row; 1985.
2. Collins JC. Good to Great: Why Some Companies Make the Leap—and Others Don't. 1st ed. New York, NY: Harper Business; 2001. p. 300.

3. Collins JC. Good to Great and the Social Sectors: Why Business Thinking Is Not the Answer. 1st ed. New York, NY: HarperCollins; 2005.
4. Jain SH. The Skills Doctors and Nurses Need to Be Effective Executives. Harv Bus Rev. 2015. Available from: https://hbr.org/2015/04/the-skills-doctors-need-to-be-effective-executives.
5. Mangrulkar RS, Saint S, Chu S, Tierney LM. What Is the Role of the Clinical "Pearl"? Am J Med. 2002;113(7):617-24.
6. Northouse PG. Leadership: Theory and practice. 8th ed. Thousand Oaks, CA: Sage publications; 2018.
7. Saint S, Krein SL, Stock RW. Preventing Hospital Infections: Real-World Problems, Realistic Solutions. New York, NY: Oxford University Press; 2015. p. 155.
8. Schlender B. New Wisdom from Steve Jobs on Technology, Hollywood, and How "Good Management Is like the Beatles." Fast Company. 2012 Apr 17.
9. Chopra V, Saint S. Leadership & Professional Development: Hire Hard, Manage Easy. J Hosp Med 2019;14:74.

RULE 2: FORGE THE FOLLOWERS YOU WANT

1. Kelley RE. In Praise of Followers. Boston, MA: Harvard Business School Press; 1988.
2. Saint S, Krein SL, Stock RW. Preventing Hospital Infections: Real-World Problems, Realistic Solutions. New York, NY: Oxford University Press; 2015. p. 155.

RULE 3: TRY A STRESS BUSTER

1. Gilmartin H, Goyal A, Hamati MC, Mann J, Saint S, Chopra V. Brief Mindfulness Practices for Healthcare Providers-a Systematic Literature Review. Am J Med. 2017;130(10):1219.e1-e17.

2. Health NIoM. 5 Things You Should Know about Stress. Available from: https://www.nimh.nih.gov/health/publications/stress/index .shtml.

3. Hougaard R, Carter J. If You Aspire to Be a Great Leader, Be Present. Harv Bus Rev. 2017. Available from: https://hbr.org/2017/12/if-you-aspire-to-be-a-great-leader-be-present.

4. Saint S, Krein SL, Stock RW. Preventing Hospital Infections: Real-World Problems, Realistic Solutions. New York, NY: Oxford University Press; 2015. p. 155.

5. Sutcliffe KM, Vogus TJ, Dane E. Mindfulness in Organizations: A Cross-Level Review. Annu Rev Organ Psychol Organ Behav. 2016;3(1):55–81.

6. Saint S, Chopra V. How Doctors Can Be Better Mentors. Harv Bus Rev. 2018. Available from: https://hbr.org/2018/10/how-doctors -can-be-better-mentors.

RULE 4: WATCH YOUR TLR

1. Goulston M. How to Know If You Talk Too Much. Harv Bus Rev. 2015. Available from: https://hbr.org/2015/06/how-to-know-if-you -talk-too-much.

2. Saint S, Chopra V. Leadership & Professional Development: Know Your TLR. J Hosp Med. 2019;14:189.

RULE 5: BEEF UP YOUR EQ

1. Barrett LF. Try These Two Smart Techniques to Help You Master Your Emotions [Internet]. 2018 [cited 2018 Jul 12]. Available from: https://ideas.ted.com/try-these-two-smart-techniques-to-help-you -master-your-emotions/.

2. Chamorro-Premuzic T. Can You Really Improve Your Emotional Intelligence? Harv Bus Rev. 2013. Available from: https://hbr.org/2013/05/can-you-really-improve-your-em.

3. Goleman D. Emotional Intelligence [Internet]. Date Unknown [cited 2018 Jul 12]. Available from: http://www.danielgoleman.info/topics/emotional-intelligence/.

4. Goleman D. Social Intelligence: The New Science of Human Relationships. New York, NY: Bantam Books; 2007.

5. Malone MS. The Secret to Midcareer Success. The Wall Street Journal. 2018 Feb 11.

6. Saint S, Krein SL, Stock RW. Preventing Hospital Infections: Real-World Problems, Realistic Solutions. New York, NY: Oxford University Press; 2015. p. 155.

RULE 6: KNOW WHEN TO BE TIGHT—OR LOOSE

1. Blanchard KH, Johnson S. The One Minute Manager. 1st Morrow ed. New York, NY: Morrow; 1982. p. 111.

2. Peters TJ, Waterman RH. In Search of Excellence: Lessons from America's Best-Run Companies. New York, NY: Warner; 1982.

RULE 7: FORGIVE AND REMEMBER

1. Bosk CL. Forgive and Remember: Managing Medical Failure. Chicago, IL: University of Chicago Press; 2003.

2. Sutton RI. Forgive and Remember: How a Good Boss Responds to Mistakes. Harv Bus Rev. 2010. Available from: https://hbr.org/2010/08/forgive-and-remember-how-a-goo.

RULE 8: DON'T FORGET YOU ARE A ROLE MODEL

1. Gewertz BL, Logan DC. Phase IV: Team President. The Best Medicine. New York, NY: Springer; 2015. p. 61-71.
2. Harrod M, Saint S. Teaching Inpatient Medicine: What Every Physician Needs to Know. New York, NY: Oxford University Press; 2017.

RULE 9: REMEMBER THE TREE-CLIMBING MONKEY

1. Halpern G. The Higher Leaders Climb, the More Others See [Internet]. 2017 [cited 2018 Jul 17]. Available from: https://aboutleaders.com/higher-leaders-climb-more-others-see.

RULE 10: COUNTER THE CONSTIPATORS

1. Saint S, Kowalski CP, Banaszak-Holl J, Forman J, Damschroder L, Krein SL. How Active Resisters and Organizational Constipators Affect Health Care-Acquired Infection Prevention Efforts. Jt Comm J Qual Patient Saf. 2009;35(5):239-46.
2. Saint S, Krein SL, Stock RW. Preventing Hospital Infections: Real-World Problems, Realistic Solutions. New York, NY: Oxford University Press; 2015. p. 155.

RULE 11: CULTIVATE EFFECTIVE MENTORS

1. Chopra V, Arora VM, Saint S. Will You Be My Mentor?—Four Archetypes to Help Mentees Succeed in Academic Medicine. JAMA Intern Med. 2018;178(2):175-6.
2. Chopra V, Saint S. 6 Things Every Mentor Should Do. Harv Bus Rev. 2017. Available from: https://hbr.org/2017/03/6-things-every-mentor-should-do.

3. Gladwell M. The Tipping Point: How Little Things Can Make a Big Difference. Boston, MA: Little, Brown; 2006.
4. Waljee JF, Chopra V, Saint S. Mentoring Millennials. JAMA. 2018;319:1547-8.
5. Saint S, Chopra V. How Doctors Can Be Better Mentors. Harv Bus Rev. 2018. Available from: https://hbr.org/2018/10/how-doctors -can-be-better-mentors.

RULE 12: DEVELOP EFFECTIVE MENTEES

1. Chopra V, Dixon-Woods M, Saint S. The Four Golden Rules of Effective Menteeship. BMJ Careers. 2016.
2. Chopra V, Saint S. What Mentors Wish Their Mentees Knew. Harv Bus Rev. 2017. Available from: https://hbr.org/2017/11/ what-mentors-wish-their-mentees-knew.
3. Vaughn V, Saint S, Chopra V. Mentee Missteps: Tales From the Academic Trenches. JAMA. 2017;317:475-6.

RULE 13: AVOID MENTORSHIP MALPRACTICE

1. CBRE. Mentoring Playbook 2017. Available from: http://elearn resources.cbre.com/TrainingandDevelopment/AMS/Mentoring _Playbook.pdf.
2. Chopra V, Edelson DP, Saint S. Mentorship Malpractice. JAMA. 2016;315(14):1453-4.

RULE 14: WRITE IT DOWN

1. Gawande A. The Checklist Manifesto: How to Get Things Right. 1st ed. New York, NY: Metropolitan Books-Henry Holt & Co; 2010. p. 209.

2. Paul A. Two Things to Do after Every Meeting. Harv Bus Rev. 2015. Available from: https://hbr.org/2015/11/two-things-to-do-after-every-meeting.

RULE 15: MAKE A FRIEND BEFORE YOU NEED ONE

1. Sandstrom GM, Dunn EW. Social Interactions and Well-Being: The Surprising Power of Weak Ties. Pers Soc Psychol Bull. 2014;40(7):910–22.

RULE 16: SMILE EARLY AND OFTEN

1. Collins JC. Good to Great and the Social Sectors: Why Business Thinking Is Not the Answer. 1st ed. New York, NY: HarperCollins; 2005. p. 35.
2. Harrod M, Saint S. Teaching Inpatient Medicine: What Every Physician Needs to Know. New York, NY: Oxford University Press; 2017.
3. Li D. What's the Science Behind a Smile? [Internet]. 2014 [cited 2018 Jul 12]. Available from: https://www.britishcouncil.org/voices-magazine/famelab-whats-science-behind-smile.

RULE 17: MOTIVATE CHANGE FROM WITHIN

1. Miller WR, Rollnick S. Motivational Interviewing: Helping People Change. 3rd ed. New York, NY: Guilford Press; 2012.
2. Saint S, Bloor L, Chopra V. Motivational Interviewing for Healthcare Providers. BMJ Opinion. 2016. Available from: http://blogs.bmj.com/bmj/2016/11/30/vineet-chopra-et-al-motivational-interviewing-for-healthcare-providers/.

RULE 18: WATCH THE CLOCK

1. Lipman V. 5 Simple Steps to More Efficient, Effective Meetings. Forbes. 2013. Available from: https://www.forbes.com/sites/victor lipman/2013/03/01/5-simple-steps-to-more-efficient-effective -meetings.

RULE 19: LET DATA SET YOU FREE

1. Meddings J, Rogers MAM, Krein SL, Fakih MG, Olmsted RN, Saint S. Reducing Unnecessary Urinary Catheter Use and Other Strategies to Prevent Catheter-Associated Urinary Tract Infection: An Integrative Review. BMJ Qual Saf. 2014;23(4):277-89.
2. Saint S, Krein SL, Stock RW. Preventing Hospital Infections: Real-World Problems, Realistic Solutions. New York, NY: Oxford University Press; 2015. p. 155.
3. Saint S, Greene MT, Krein SL, et al. A Program to Prevent Catheter-Associated Urinary Tract Infection in Acute Care. N Engl J Med 2016;374:2111-9.

RULE 20: EMBRACE DIFFICULT CONVERSATIONS

1. Stone D, Heen S, Patton B. Difficult Conversations: How to Discuss What Matters Most. New York, NY: Penguin; 2010.
2. Welch J, Welch S. Winning. New York, NY: Harper Business; 2005.

RULE 21: ENCOURAGE DISAGREEMENT; DISCOURAGE CONFLICT

1. Brett J, Goldberg SB. How to Handle a Disagreement on Your Team. Harv Bus Rev. 2017. Available from: https://hbr.org/2017/ 07/how-to-handle-a-disagreement-on-your-team.

2. Love S. The Case for Encouraging Disagreement. LinkedIn. 2017. Available from: https://www.linkedin.com/pulse/case-encouraging -disagreement-shawnee-love.
3. Mill JS. On Liberty. 1st ed. London, England: John W. Parker and Son; 1859.
4. Roth D. Supporting Healthy Conflict in the Workplace. Forbes. 2013. Available from: https://www.forbes.com/sites/davidroth/2013/ 07/29/supporting-healthy-conflict-in-the-workplace.

RULE 22: POSITIVE DEVIANCE IS YOUR FRIEND

1. Bryant A. How to Be a C.E.O., from a Decade's Worth of Them. The New York Times. 2017 Oct 27.
2. Cameron KS, Dutton JE, Quinn RE. Positive Organizational Scholarship: Foundations of a New Discipline. 1st ed. San Francisco, CA: Berrett-Koehler; 2003. p. 465.
3. Katzenberg J. The Benefit of a Boot Out the Door. The New York Times. 2009 Nov 7.

RULE 23: USE STRESS TO ENHANCE PERFORMANCE

1. Harrod M, Saint S. Teaching Inpatient Medicine: What Every Physician Needs to Know. New York, NY: Oxford University Press; 2017.

RULE 24: YOU CREATE THE CULTURE

1. Gruenert S, Whitaker T. School Culture Rewired: How to Define, Assess, and Transform It. Alexandria, VA: ASCD; 2015.
2. Walter E. Thoughtful Branding: Where the Company Begins and Ends. Forbes. 2013. Available from: https://www.forbes.com/ sites/ekaterinawalter/2013/09/24/thoughtful-branding-where-the -company-begins-and-ends.

3. Williams Jr. GS. (Informal) Leadership. LinkedIn. 2015. Available from: https://www.linkedin.com/pulse/informal-leadership-garr-s -williams-jr-.

RULE 25: PURSUE PROFOUND SIMPLICITY

1. Emerson RW, Emerson EW. The Complete Works of Ralph Waldo Emerson: Representative Men [Vol. 4]. Boston, MA: Houghton Mifflin Company; 1903.
2. Schutz W. Profound Simplicity. London, England: Turnstone Books; 1979.

RULE 26: KNOW WHEN AND WHERE TO DRAW THE LINE

1. Dahl M. Why Office Friendships Can Feel So Awkward. The New York Times. 2018 May 28.
2. Schawbel D. Dr. Henry Cloud: How to Manage Boundaries in the Workplace. Forbes. 2013. Available from: https://www.forbes.com/ sites/danschawbel/2013/05/10/dr-henry-cloud-how-to-manage -boundaries-in-the-workplace.
3. Welch J, Welch S. Winning. New York, NY: Harper Business; 2005.
4. Zetlin M. When Trouble at Home Becomes Trouble in the Office. Inc. 2013. Available from: https://www.inc.com/minda-zetlin/employee -facing-personal-problems-heres-what-to-do.html.

RULE 27: PATIENCE IS A VIRTUE

1. Kouzes JM, Posner BZ. Learning Leadership: The Five Fundamentals of Becoming an Exemplary Leader. Hoboken, NJ: Wiley; 2016.

2. Gordon S. Nursing Against the Odds: How Healthcare Cost Cutting, Media Stereotypes, and Medical Hubris Undermine Nurses and Patient Care. Ithaca, NY: Cornell University Press; 2005.

RULE 28: NEGOTIATE WITH THE END IN MIND

1. Fisher R, Ury WL, Patton B. Getting to Yes: Negotiating Agreement without Giving In. 2nd ed. New York, NY: Penguin; 1991. p. 200.

RULE 29: DON'T FORGET FAMILY

1. Saunders EG. What to Do When Personal and Professional Commitments Compete for Your Time. Harv Bus Rev. 2018. Available from: https://hbr.org/2018/04/what-to-do-when-when-personal-and -professional-commitments-compete-for-your-time.
2. Weber L, Lublin JS. The Daddy Juggle: Work, Life, Family and Chaos. The Wall Street Journal. 2014 Jun 12.
3. Yoder SK, Yoder IS, Yoder L. Work, Family and the Problem of Balance. The Wall Street Journal. 2010 Jan 17.

RULE 30: LEAD WITH KINDNESS, COMPASSION, AND LOVE

1. Bennis W, Nanus B. The Strategies for Taking Charge. New York, NY: Harper Row; 1985.
2. Donabedian A. A Founder of Quality Assessment Encounters a Troubled System Firsthand. Interview by Fitzhugh Mullan. Health Affairs. 2001;20(1):137.
3. Williams R. Why We Need Kind and Compassionate Leaders. Financial Post. 2012 Sep 13.

ABOUT THE AUTHORS

Dr. Sanjay Saint is the Chief of Medicine at the VA Ann Arbor Healthcare System and the George Dock Professor of Internal Medicine at the University of Michigan. His research focuses on patient safety, leadership, and medical decision-making. He has authored over 350 peer-reviewed papers in major medical journals including nearly 100 in the New England Journal of Medicine or JAMA. He has also written for The Wall Street Journal, Harvard Business Review, and other major news outlets and has published numerous books. He received the Mark Wolcott Award from the Department of Veterans Affairs as the National VA Physician of the Year in 2016, and a major mentorship award from the University of Michigan Health System in 2018. He has given invited lectures on leadership, followership, and change management throughout the world.

Dr. Vineet Chopra is the Chief of the Division of Hospital Medicine, an Associate Professor of Internal Medicine at the University of Michigan, and a Research Scientist at the VA Ann Arbor Healthcare System. Dr. Chopra's research focuses on improving the safety of hospitalized patients through the prevention of hospital-acquired complications. He is the recipient of numerous teaching and research awards including the 2016 Kaiser Permanente Award for Clinical Teaching and has published over 200 peer-reviewed articles in major medical journals. He has also written numerous articles in the Harvard Business Review, JAMA, and the British Medical Journal on mentorship.

ABOUT THE ARTIST

Victoria Bornstein is a painter, illustrator, and graphic designer based in Chicago, IL. She received her Bachelors in Art and Design from the University of Michigan in 2018, has since then worked in the Education Department at the Museum of Fine Arts, Boston, and is now a graphic designer at OrgStory in Chicago. When not at work, she is in her studio painting, hiking, discovering new artists on Instagram, hanging with friends and family, or doodling on any piece of paper she can get her hands on!

For more of Victoria Bornstein's work, please visit her website here: https://www.victoriabornstein.com

CPSIA information can be obtained
at www.ICGtesting.com
Printed in the USA
BVHW052252300619
552337BV00001B/2/P

9 781607 855415